DAY SURGERY
A Handbook for Nurses

~~~ICAL LIBRARY
~~~FORD POSTGRADUATE
~~~ICAL CENTRE
WATFORD GENERAL HOSPITAL
VICARAGE ROAD
WATFORD WD1 8HB

DAY SURGERY
A Handbook for Nurses

Elizabeth Sutherland
Royal Victoria Infirmary
and Associated Hospitals NHS Trust,
Newcastle upon Tyne,
UK

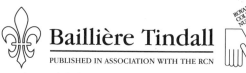

Baillière Tindall

PUBLISHED IN ASSOCIATION WITH THE RCN

London   Philadelphia   Toronto   Sydney   Tokyo

Baillière Tindall   24–28 Oval Road
London NW1 7DX

The Curtis Center
Independence Square West
Philadelphia, PA 19106-3399, USA

Harcourt Brace & Company
55 Horner Avenue
Toronto, Ontario, M8Z 4X6, Canada

Harcourt Brace & Company, Australia
30-52 Smidmore Street
Marrickville
NSW 2204, Australia

Harcourt Brace & Company, Japan
Ichibancho Central Building
22-1 Ichibancho
Chiyoda-ku, Tokyo 102, Japan

© 1996 D. E. Sutherland

The right of D. E. Sutherland to be identified as the author of this
work has been asserted by her in accordance with the
Copyright, Designs and Patents Act 1988.

Cover photo reproduced by kind permission of Christine Hudson.

This book is printed on acid-free paper

All rights reserved. No part of this publication may be reproduced,
stored in a retrieval system or transmitted, in any form or by any other
means, electronic, mechanical, photocopying or otherwise, without the
prior permission of Baillière Tindall, 24-28 Oval Road, London NW1 7DX

A catalogue record for this book is available from the British Library

ISBN 0-7020-1988-7

Typeset by Florencetype Ltd, Stoodleigh, Devon

Printed and bound in Great Britain by
WBC Book Manufacturers, Bridgend, Glamorgan

Contents

Preface

This handbook is intended to provide nurses with a comprehensive, step-by-step guide to day surgical nursing and day care for the increasing number of patients who, nowadays, undergo numerous day surgery procedures, day treatments and diagnostic tests within acute hospital settings.

It is clear that nursing in today's NHS is becoming much more demanding. The nursing profession is being asked to balance organisational and management skills with more effective and efficient methods of delivering nursing care. This is particularly the case in day surgery where efficient organisation and planning are as crucial to success as is the patient's undoubted need for nursing support and guidance.

This handbook is an attempt to balance some of the most important practical steps and day-to-day solutions for managing day surgery combined with the best possible care for the growing number of patients who spend very little time in contact with health professionals. Day case patients have, after all, the same needs as their in-patient counterparts but they also have additional information needs. They and their families need to know that someone will provide them with enough knowledge to be able to care for themselves within a very short time after their surgical intervention.

The author, who spent ten years developing the role of the nurse in day surgery, recognised that many nurses were being expected to take on a wider role as the prime organisers in their day surgery facilities. It became clear that there was also a need for nurses to support each other and share their experiences. As a founder member of the Royal College of Nursing's Special Interest Group for Day Surgery Nurses, the author is committed to supporting nurses in a very different and difficult field. The Day Surgery Special Interest Group has had considerable success so far with a fast growing (free!) membership and has run two very well attended Autumn conferences in the last two years.

The British Association of Day Surgery, an organisation committed to a multi-disciplinary approach to care with a membership of nurses, surgeons and anaesthetists, has also been very active in promoting day surgery through its conferences and journal. (See Appendix for further information.)

A definitive textbook on day surgery nursing may in the future better fulfil the need to address the "theory – practice gap" in what may eventually be called Ambulatory Care. The author saw the need to fill a gap, however, by providing day surgery nurses with a working handbook and this text is not intended to provide an in depth examination of background theory. It does, however, offer a framework for nursing, based upon nursing theory, and is designed to ensure that day surgery nursing remains, and continues to develop, as a successful service, contributing to ensuring that each experience is a positive one for this ever-growing number of day patients.

The logical layout of each chapter, with a number of checklists and examples of protocols and documentation, is intended to be an easy and readable guide for all nurses who care for any patients who spend very little time in their care. Each chapter is designed to reinforce the fact that day care can only be successful within a well-planned organisation and with prepared, educated and committed nursing staff, caring for well-informed and normally self-caring patients.

It is important to realise, too, that nurses do not always care for day cases in a purpose-built discrete day surgery unit. Patients for short stay surgery, endoscopy day cases, programmed investigations and out-patient interventions are all to be found in traditional medical or surgical wards, out-patient and X-ray departments and clinics. There is a need to guarantee a multi-disciplinary approach to the management of all such patients, with the main objective of developing quality day case treatment wherever it may take place.

Increasingly many of the medical journals are addressing the issues of short stay surgery, out-patient anaesthesia and the newer, less invasive surgical techniques. Nursing journals will want to match this interest as more and more patients are cared for as day patients, frequently now outside the acute hospital setting. The author hopes that this short handbook will encourage nurses caring for day cases to submit their own experiences for publication so that this new discipline can build a greater body of knowledge upon which to base day case practice.

The author would like to thank all those who have provided inspiration and support, particularly one of the principal pioneers of modern day surgical anaesthesia, Dr Tom Ogg, and all those who have remained patient and understanding towards what, it is hoped, will be a successful project and a useful tool for nurses working in a dynamic and important form of nursing care.

Elizabeth Sutherland
Newcastle, July 1996

1

The Background to Day Surgery

What is day surgery? – Building a quality service – Some definitions – The growth of day surgery – The shifting emphasis in health care – The unique needs of day patients – The unique features of day surgical care – The nurse's role in organising day surgery – The scope of this handbook

THIS CHAPTER: Defines day surgery and briefly examines its growth and development. It sets day surgery in the context of health care today and suggests that there are some unique needs surrounding the provision of a quality service to day patients.

WHAT IS DAY SURGERY?

A basic definition of day surgery is the care and treatment of patients who are admitted for a planned day surgical procedure. They are discharged on the same day and require a bed or trolley for a period of recovery prior to discharge.

Day patients may undergo a number of minor and intermediate procedures and can be cared for in a variety of settings. Although the ideal place for day surgery may be the integrated day surgery unit with its own operating theatre and primary and secondary recovery facilities, there are still significant numbers of day cases on day wards, conventional wards, in endoscopy rooms and X-ray departments.

Nursing care for day patients should be no less important than for their in-patient counterparts but where there is competition for care between acutely ill in-patients and day patients it will be easy to guess who might lose out! For this reason the integrated day unit which caters solely for these patients and which has a dedicated staff catering for day patients and their unique information needs will be the preferred option.

Any definition of what constitutes a suitable case for day surgery will fluctuate according to clinical decisions made by individual surgeons. As surgical techniques improve or change, many operations which are not considered suitable at present, may become feasible for day surgery. The Royal College of Surgeons published lists of suitable procedures in their report in 1992, but these were by no means comprehensive and have already altered and expanded radically in recent years.

BUILDING A QUALITY SERVICE

Many health care professionals have been slow to acknowledge the value of a structured and efficient organisation, specifically equipped and designed to ensure that day patients can progress safely, without complication, through each day surgical episode.

Since this is a relatively unfamiliar form of treatment, the public may still need to be persuaded of its benefits. Therefore, all day surgery treatment must be developed as a high quality service which can demonstrate measurable benefits for patients. If this cannot be achieved it will be seen, quite justifiably, as an inferior alternative to in-patient treatment.

Also, since day surgery is a relatively new concept to many people it is likely that a poor quality day surgical service will attract adverse publicity. Despite everyone's best efforts, the public may perceive this form of treatment as a cheap option or a government ploy to reduce costs. Patients and their families may also view this 'new' form of treatment with heightened anxiety. They could feel that they are being deprived of conventional in-patient care with a recovery period in hospital and that they will have to fend for themselves at home with no advice or support if things go wrong.

To counteract what are very real concerns about 'same day treatment', priority must be given to incorporating systems and methods into the process which can guarantee the safety of day surgery treatment.

Efficiency, skilled technique and a predictable and uneventful recovery from surgery become increasingly important if patients are to recover safely in their own homes. Day patients must experience fewer, or none, of the side effects which have traditionally been alleviated by timely intervention from an experienced nurse during a night spent under observation on a surgical ward. If patients do develop minor post-operative symptoms, they must know what to expect and they must be provided with the knowledge and ability to deal with these problems themselves.

There should, therefore, be a continuous programme of measurement, specifically designed to determine the effect of surgical and anaesthetic techniques on the recovery of day patients. It is equally important to determine whether the patients are satisfied before consistency of outcome can be properly reported.

SOME DEFINITIONS

Box 1.1 lists some common definitions which will be used throughout this handbook. These definitions will be familiar to most nurses who have experience in caring for day cases, but they may help to clarify some of the main concepts for those who are unfamiliar with day case surgery.

Box 1.1 **Important definitions**

The day surgery patient: A planned admission, admitted for a planned day surgical procedure, discharged on the same day and needing to occupy a bed or trolley for a period of recovery prior to discharge.

A day surgical case: Any surgical procedure from which the patient can safely recover at home with minimal post-operative observation or further post-operative treatment.

There should be minimal risk of post-operative haemorrhage, uncontrollable pain or major post-operative complications.

The 'ward attender': A patient who may attend a surgical ward for treatment or dressings, post-operative checks by their surgeon, or for advice from ward staff.

The out-patient: A patient who may receive minor treatment in an out-patient department, who will usually walk in and out and who requires little or no recovery time.

The integrated or dedicated day surgery unit: A facility, adapted or purpose-built, catering solely for the treatment of day surgical cases. The unit contains admission, anaesthetic, operating and recovery facilities and is staffed by dedicated day surgery nursing staff. There may or may not be facilities for endoscopy and medical diagnostic procedures. These units often maintain and manage their own waiting lists.

The day ward: A ward which caters solely for day cases and utilises existing operating theatres within a main theatre complex. Patients may be incorporated into in-patient theatre lists, or lists made up solely of day cases. Frequently other patients may be treated on day wards who require dressings, suture removal or other diagnostic procedures.

The surgical ward: Hospitals which do not possess integrated day surgery units or day wards still care for their day patients in surgical wards. Patients may be admitted directly from a common waiting list which incorporates both in-patient and day cases. They will frequently be treated within a routine in-patient theatre list. This, perhaps, is the least efficient method for day surgery care since greater demands may be placed on nursing time by acutely ill in-patients.

THE GROWTH OF DAY SURGERY

There is nothing very new about treating people as day cases. Patients have frequently undergone minor surgical treatment and been discharged to recover at home on the same day. Indeed, only a few years ago, it was far from uncommon, for some procedures, such as tonsillectomy, to be carried out in people's own homes.

It could be said that the birth of day surgery in this country took place in Glasgow, at the beginning of this century. Thousands of paediatric surgical procedures were treated as day cases. Nicoll (1909) believed that this was a far less traumatic way to treat children who were already suffering from osteomyelitis and a variety of congenital orthopaedic anomalies. He performed minor orthopaedic procedures on these children as day cases and immediately returned them to their mothers' arms, allowing them home to recover in familiar surroundings.

After Nicoll described his treatment of these children there was no immediate explosion of day surgery. It was slow to evolve, at least in this country, and for many years surgeons continued to tread warily. Some considered that it was unsafe and unfair to patients to be left to their own devices so soon after surgery (Cassie 1973).

While purpose-built facilities for day surgery have been slow to evolve in the UK (and there are still large numbers of day cases going through more conventional surgical areas), a revolution has been taking place in the USA.

In the early 1960s a number of day surgery facilities throughout the USA were converted from existing surgical facilities, notably at the University of California and George Washington University. These became research-based day surgery centres, and were particularly important in the development of modern anaesthesia (Smith & White 1994). As a result of the dissemination of this research the advantages of day surgery were closely examined and began to be emulated elsewhere. Day Surgery facilities, therefore, began to appear in most public hospitals and the system was gradually adopted within both public and private health care facilities.

A free-standing 'Ambulatory Surgi-center' was established in Phoenix, Arizona in 1969 and was able to attract experienced anaesthetists and nurses to support efficient scheduling and more productive use of the surgeon's time. The centre demonstrated improvement in patient flow and became a cost-effective, marketable and efficient facility in which to treat day patients (Reed & Ford 1974). Facilities such as these became more popular. Often they are not attached or even close to acute general hospitals, but served remote communities, delivering minor surgical treatment closer to patients' own homes.

'Same-day' treatment for minor and intermediate surgical conditions therefore became the norm throughout the USA. An important factor which contributed to this growth and popularity was the high cost of in-patient care. Patients who pay for their own treatment, or who might face higher insurance premiums as a consequence of treatment, will usually opt to have their treatment on a day-case basis.

Indeed, because most people in the USA are responsible for contributing to their own medical insurance, there is an obvious economic advantage in day surgical treatment. This concept has been developed to such a degree that, even for major surgery such as vaginal hysterectomy, some medical insurance companies will reimburse only a 23-hour hospital stay (still a day case) for a normally fit, healthy individual.

Despite modern improvements in anaesthesia and surgical technique, it is debatable whether day surgery would have been adopted as enthusiastically in this country, because private medical insurance is still not the norm. The catalyst for expansion came from rising waiting lists and escalating National Health Service costs. These factors led to a scrutiny of and consequent reduction in the numbers of in-patient beds and a shift from acute care towards community and primary care, designed to prevent prolonged hospital stays.

There has, therefore been a significant increase in the number of patients undergoing day surgery in the UK during the last decade, as shown in Fig. 1.1. It is generally accepted that this growth has occurred as a direct consequence of escalating costs in health care and long surgical waiting lists. Further impetus came from the

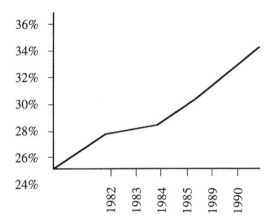

Fig. 1.1   Day case admissions; Surgical acute day cases as a percentage of all elective surgical admissions. (From **Day Surgery**, A Task Force Report, NHS Management Executive, 1993)

need to realise government targets encapsulated in the Patient's Charter (Department of Health, 1995). Thus, government has actively encouraged innovative ways to deliver a safe and effective service for the ever-increasing number of day surgery patients.

THE SHIFTING EMPHASIS IN HEALTH CARE

The significant growth of surgical day care in the last ten years has therefore been due to changed government imperatives in health care. Health services were challenged to demonstrate value for money by better utilisation of expensive in-patient beds, while simultaneously reducing the number of patients awaiting surgical treatment. Many of the considerable advances in surgical technique and the pharmaceutical advances in anaesthesia might never have occurred unless these factors had had to be addressed by every health authority.

The evolution and expansion of day case surgery was not, until recently, subject to the same financial imperatives in the UK as in the USA. However, in the last decade, government directives and recommendations have set specific targets for health

Box 1.2 **Publications supporting the growth of day surgery**

Guidelines for Day Case Surgery, Royal College of Surgeons (first published 1985, revised 1992)

■ Sets out the RCS view of the scope of day surgery and facilities required. It encouraged surgeons and health authorities to develop the service.

A Short Cut To Better Services, Audit Commission (1990)

■ Identified some of the obstacles to the growth of day surgery in England and Wales and suggested ways to overcome these which would also maintain and improve standards of patient care.

Day Surgery – Making it happen, The Value for Money Unit, NHSME (1992)

■ Identified the benefits of treating patients as day cases rather than occupying in-patient beds. Examined the critical success factors for setting up day surgery and encouraged hospitals to adopt measures which make greater use of such facilities.

**Day Surgery – Report by the Day Surgery Task Force, NHS Management Executive (1993)

■ Examined strategies for the expansion of day surgery – ways of achieving higher targets; information and data collection issues; training and education; quality, audit and standard setting

Just for the Day – Children admitted to Hospital for Day Treatment, Rosemary Thornes, NAWCH (1991)

■ Emphasised the careful planning required for day treatment for children. Provided a managerial tool to help hospitals to improve the quality of their care for this group of patients.

Day Case Surgery for Cataract, Scottish Health Service Advisory Council, NHSME Scotland (1992)

■ Recommended good practice and appropriate systems for the management of ophthalmic day case services.

Day Case Surgery with Special Reference to the Elderly, Working Group on Acute Beds and the Elderly, Scottish Office (1993)

■ Considered the effect of the increasing elderly population on the use of acute hospital in-patient facilities and found that elderly patients should not be excluded from day case surgery on chronological rather than biological grounds. Advocated the provision of patient hotels for this group of patients.

Patient Hotels – A Quality Alternative to Ward Care, The Value for Money Unit, NHSME (1992)

■ Examined the potential benefits and constraints of accommodating suitable patients in a patient hotel as an alternative to a hospital ward.

authorities to increase the proportion of their day cases and have generally advocated the development of day surgery facilities as a means of reducing the number of acute beds.

Reports issued by the Audit Commission (1990), the Value for Money Unit (1992) and the NHS Management Executive Task Force (1993) also supported the growth of day surgery. (See Box 1.2.) These reports, along with other publications, maintain that day surgery should increase not only for financial reasons but because, at best, it could bring positive benefits for patients, such as ease of access, convenience and a better quality service.

THE UNIQUE NEEDS OF DAY PATIENTS

For most nurses, caring for day case patients on a general, surgical ward is not a remarkable or even an unusual occurrence. Day patients have, however, often been considered a low priority (Morgan & Reynolds 1991). These patients may often become unwelcome additions to an already busy work load for those caring for more acutely ill patients. For this reason, day patients were traditionally allocated to the care of the most junior nurse and often operated on by the houseman, senior house officer or junior registrar.

When asked day patients frequently say that they receive inadequate information about how they will feel, what to do and what to expect from their treatment (Audit Commission 1991).

The very nature of day surgery implies that patients have minimal contact with health professionals. It must be important, therefore, that strategies are developed which will provide patients with a working knowledge of what to do and what to expect during their treatment. If they are to prepare and to care for themselves they must be given some sense of control in the whole process.

THE UNIQUE FEATURES OF DAY SURGICAL CARE

Achieving high-quality day surgery nursing practice will not be concerned solely with acquiring basic competence in peri-operative nursing, operating theatre or recovery technique. Day surgery nurses need to understand the greater psychological and informational needs of day patients.

See
Chapter 6

It has certainly not been universally recognised that 'peri-operative nursing' and good quality care for day patients warrants more refined skills, experience and competence than that acquired from the basic, rudimentary training of both nurses and doctors. Day surgery nursing is becoming a specialism in its own right, as Morgan and Reynolds recognised in 1991.

Health service managers have only fairly recently acknowledged the important role that nurses can fulfil in day surgery. Slowly they are beginning to realise that, in order to ensure a well-designed, functioning day surgery facility, they must employ nursing staff of sufficiently high calibre, with the ability to make a significant contribution to all the components within the day surgery service. Chapter 6 will expand on the competencies which nurses will need to attain to achieve maximum effectiveness in day surgical practice.

See Chapter 6

Day Surgery is a legitimate specialism in nursing because of the importance of the informational and educational aspects of care in this area. Managers will also recognise that the needs of day patients are unique in this respect. To address these needs they will wish to employ personnel who can provide more than a mere blend of theatre, recovery and surgical nursing care.

Chapter 5 discusses possible strategies for designing information which will equip patients with enough knowledge to avoid unpleasant and unexpected surprises during their recovery at home. It is important that nurses should begin to challenge the assumptions that many health professionals make about the amount of information patients need. They often believe that by censoring or providing only the minimal amount of information that patients will be spared unnecessary anxiety.

See Chapter 5

THE NURSE'S ROLE IN ORGANISING DAY SURGERY

Throughout the following chapters, it will be stressed that good organisation is the key to efficient working practices in a dynamic and fast-moving area such as day surgery.

Good organisation, clear definition and minute attention to formulating unambiguous, shared protocols for nursing day surgery patients will help to secure high quality care for patients who spend only the briefest of periods in contact with the system. Because of the need for psychosocial support during the short time these patients spend in contact with health professionals, it will be important to employ nurses who are skilled communicators with highly developed interpersonal skills.

Much of what follows in subsequent chapters might appear relatively simplistic to the experienced nurse. However, whatever the level of experience there can be no harm in re-examining some of the ways in which practical skills can be built upon good theoretical nursing practice. Good nursing care in day surgery, therefore, must be based upon a well-organised process with the emphasis firmly placed upon comprehensive assessment, good selection, education and a high level of support and guidance for an ever-growing number of patients and their families.

THE SCOPE OF THIS HANDBOOK

This handbook is designed, not to provide all the answers, but as a guide for nurses who care for day patients, in whatever setting, and to help them to understand the special needs of these patients. It is not intended solely for nurses who work in an integrated or dedicated day unit.

It may be relevant to apply the standards and principles outlined in this handbook to all short-stay patients. Patients share similar needs regardless of whether they are attending X-ray departments, programmed medical investigation units, for chemotherapy, haematology or haemodialysis treatments. This is because they also need to be provided with enough knowledge to prepare themselves for treatment and must fend for themselves when they go home.

Further reading

BRADSHAW, E.G. & Davenport, H.T. (1989) **Day Care Surgery, Anaesthesia and Management**. Edward Arnold, London. As the title implies, this publication dwells more on day case anaesthesia but contains a chapter on the organisation of day surgery from a nursing perspective.

BURN, J.M.B. (1979) A blueprint for day surgery *Anaesthesia* **34**, pp. 790–805. A synopsis of the basic requirements for setting up a day surgery unit.

DAVIS, J.E. & DETMER, D.E. (1972) The Ambulatory Surgery Unit, *Annals of Surgery* **175** (6) pp. 857–862. Describes the early years of working in one of the first freestanding units in Phoenix, Arizona.

DEPARTMENT OF HEALTH (1995) **The Patient's Charter and You**, NHS Patient's Charter Unit. NHSME, Leeds. A reminder of the quality of care which patients are urged to expect from the health services.

ROYAL COLLEGE OF SURGEONS OF ENGLAND (1985) **Guidelines for Day Care Surgery**. Royal College of Surgeons of England, London. A useful reference guide to the early recommendations from the Royal College of Surgeons. A helpful publication to evaluate how far day surgery has progressed in a decade.

NICHOLS, K.A. (1984) **Psychological Care in Physical Illness**. Croom Helm, Kent. A practical guide, containing illuminating case studies, intended for those wishing to develop their skills in psychological care.

WHITWAM J.G. (ed.) (1994) **Day-Case Anaesthesia and Sedation**. Blackwell Scientific Publications, London. Provides clear clinical guidelines and contains some systematic studies and audits of activity in the field, mainly of anaesthesia. Also contains a chapter on nursing and unit organisation.

References

AUDIT COMMISSION (1990) **A Short Cut to Better Services**. HMSO, London.

AUDIT COMMISSION (1991) **Measuring Quality: The Patient's View of Day Surgery**, NHS Occasional Papers No. 3: HMSO, London.

CASSIE, A. (1973) Surgery in day patients. *British Medical Journal* **1** p. 542.

MORGAN, M. & REYNOLDS A. (1991) Day surgery units: Are they attractive to nurses? *Advances in Health and Nursing Care*.**1**:2, pp. 59–74.

NHS MANAGEMENT EXECUTIVE (1993) **Day Surgery**, report by the Day Surgery Task Force. HMSO, London.

NICOLL, J.H. (1909) The surgery of infancy (ii). *British Medical Journal:* pp. 753–754.

REED, W.A. & FORD, J.A. (1974) The Surgicenter: An ambulatory facility. *Clinical Obstetrics & Gynaecology* **17** pp. 217–230.

ROYAL COLLEGE OF SURGEONS (1992) **Guidelines for Day Case Surgery**. Royal College of Surgeons of England, London.

SMITH, I. & WHITE, P.F. (1994) History and Scope of Day-Case Anaesthesia: Past, Present and Future. **Day-Case Anaesthesia and Sedation** (ed. J.G. Whitwam). Blackwell Scientific Publications, London.

SCOTTISH HEALTH SERVICE ADVISORY COUNCIL (1992) **Day Case Surgery for Cataract**. NHS Management Executive/The Scottish Office.

THORNES, R. (1991) **Just for the Day – Children admitted to hospital for day treatment**. NAWCH, London.

VALUE FOR MONEY UNIT (1991) **Day Surgery – Making it Happen**. NHS Management Executive. HMSO, London.

VALUE FOR MONEY UNIT (1992) **Patient Hotels – A Quality Alternative to Ward Care**. HMSO, London.

2

The Organisation and Management of Day Surgery

Introduction – Some of the barriers to successful day surgery management – Setting up a day surgery unit: the operational policy – The nurse as manager and coordinator of day surgery – Protocols for efficient management of day surgery

THIS CHAPTER: Discusses the role of the manager of an integrated day surgery unit, who is usually a nurse. It suggests the need for working to clear protocols, split-second timing, rigorous selection procedures and detailed planning throughout all aspects of a day patient's journey. This chapter is intended as a guide to preparing protocols and formulating operational policies as an efficient management framework for a day surgery facility.

INTRODUCTION

Following the publication of the first edition of their *Guidelines for Day Surgery* (1985), the Royal College of Surgeons advocated wider scope for day case surgery. The NHS increased the momentum by encouraging health authorities and hospitals to meet higher targets of surgical patients who could be treated as day cases. It was suggested that in many, but not all, surgical specialities at least 50–60% of surgery would become suitable for day case surgery (Royal College of Surgeons 1985).

The advent of the internal market gave 'purchasing' responsibility to health authorities and general practitioner (GP) fundholders. These purchasers use a contracting process to buy higher proportions of day surgical cases from providers. Therefore, encouraged by government policy, purchasers of health care came to expect that, if properly managed, day surgery would improve throughput and would become a more efficient and cost-effective method of reducing waiting lists and lengths of hospital stays.

See
Chapter 1

Chapter 1 discussed the fact that day cases are frequently treated in many places all over the hospital. It was assumed that there would be a more efficient service if these day cases were to be concentrated in one purpose-built facility wherever possible.

A dedicated day surgery facility, with integral theatre/s and primary and secondary recovery zones, was considered the preferred option for the increased number of patients expected. Resources did not, however, always support this ideal solution. Therefore, day wards were frequently converted from existing in-patient facilities and these continued to feed into existing in-patient theatres.

For greater throughput and efficiency, the Audit Commission (1990) advocated an independently staffed facility and, where possible, integral theatres and primary and secondary recovery areas. The Royal College of Surgeons (1992) also stressed the need for a strong team to manage such facilities. This, they suggested, should consist of a committed clinician, a business manager and a nurse manager, who would provide day-to-day management of the day surgery unit.

SOME OF THE BARRIERS TO SUCCESSFUL DAY SURGERY MANAGEMENT

Many managers and a number of clinicians were not fully prepared for the changes in working practices nor for the considerable impact that the development of day surgery could have on the whole organisation of health care provision.

Even though health providers have been encouraged to meet higher day surgery targets, universal recognition of the positive benefits of increased day surgery has been slow to materialise. There is still some difference of opinion on whether targets of 60% (of all surgery treated as day cases) can be realistically achieved. A report from the Welsh Health Planning Forum estimates that there are a number of factors, including the need for adequate social and community support, which would suggest a more reasonable target of between 40% and 50% (Dobson 1994).

The Value for Money Unit (1991), suggested that there were a significant number of people who should have been suitable for day cases but were still not being treated as such. The Audit Commission (1990) found that there were some crucial factors which militated against rapid development of day surgery. Some of these are listed below.

- **Inaccurate recording of day cases** – to identify actual numbers of day cases being treated.

- **Varying definitions about what a day case is** – where some out-patient procedures are counted as day cases.

- **Lack of specialist facilities** – lack of dedicated day surgery facilities; some hospitals also have geographical problems with theatres some distance from day wards.

- **Inefficient use of existing facilities** – mixing of emergencies, in-patients and day cases on in-patient lists, or inefficient scheduling of day case lists.

- **Poor management and organisation** – lack of pre-assessment, enforcement of selection protocols, discharge criteria and information to patients.

- **Clinician preferences for more traditional approaches** – routine or low priority and status of day surgery, loss of in-patient facilities.

- **Managers' disincentives for change** – difficulties in influencing clinical judgement; over-achieving on contracts if increasing numbers of day cases are treated.

Many people remain comfortable with their local arrangements where in-patients and day patients are treated in the same wards and on the same operating lists. Some of the arguments used to retain the status quo, also mentioned in the Audit Commission report, centred on the fact that clinicians could ensure that their in-patient beds remained occupied, and that they were able to use their minor surgery to teach their junior colleagues during their scheduled lists in in-patient theatres.

Since the NHS is committed to increasing day surgery it is important to demonstrate the benefits of well-organised day surgery. Perhaps the most effective way to do this is to show sound operational and managerial competence, to support a highly skilled, dedicated team working towards consistently successful results.

SETTING UP A DAY SURGERY UNIT: THE OPERATIONAL POLICY

Solving the problems identified in the Audit Commission report (see above) might be a reasonable starting point when organising the work of a new, or existing, day surgery facility.

Methods for data collection, working practice protocols and policies, selection guidelines, pre-assessment screening and discharge criteria should be addressed jointly by the management team. It has frequently been the case that many existing practices and procedures have evolved merely in response to the effects of unfavourable outcomes and not always as a result of planned research and rigorous evaluation. Therefore, at the outset, all protocols, policies and guidelines should be defined explicitly and developed as a framework for a pro-active operational policy.

THE NURSE AS MANAGER AND COORDINATOR OF DAY SURGERY

As co-ordinators of patient care, nurses are aware of the need to take account of the unique needs of patients in all settings. As they become experienced in day surgery, they will gain a broader understanding of the special and differing needs of day patients compared to their in-patient counterparts. As the day-to-day manager, the senior nurse plays a key role in the development,

Box 2.1   **Protocols for efficient management of day surgery**

- Pre-operative selection protocols
- Protocol for suitable procedures for day surgery
- Pre-operative screening protocol
- Protocol for providing information to patients and carers about their roles
- Scheduling and timing protocols
- Recovery and pain control protocols
- Discharge protocols

co-ordination and evaluation of team working-practices and the outcome of care within the day surgery facility.

Box 2.1 identifies some of the more important day surgery protocols specifically relevant to the needs of day patients. These will form a large part of a framework for good practice within the day surgery facility. It will usually be the role of the nurse manager to ensure that all these protocols are made explicit and that they are incorporated into the practice of every member of the team.

Many of the following protocols can be developed by nurses, in consultation with the multi-disciplinary team, and will be tailored to suit individual local conditions and the relevant trust organisational policies. They must, however, always recognise the specific requirements of day case patients.

PROTOCOLS FOR EFFICIENT MANAGEMENT OF DAY SURGERY

Pre-operative selection protocols

In the early days, nurse managers rarely contributed to policy decisions about which patients were or were not suitable for day surgery. Initially, few surgeons recognised the enormous benefits of a rigorous selection process. They certainly did not feel entirely comfortable about devolving their own decisions for suitable selection, or for the scheduling and organisation of their day case lists, to nurses.

However, it was not always feasible, in a busy out-patient department, to assess suitability and gain a holistic view of each prospective day patient. For this reason nurses began to advocate an in-depth pre-assessment of all day surgery patients as a legitimate extension to their role.

As well as assessing a patient's physical suitability for day surgery, it is important to determine the social circumstances and psychological status of day patients. Their perceptions about what constitutes suitable treatment from the NHS may also need to be determined.

Anaesthetists, who are specifically concerned with the general physical status of day surgery candidates, initially advocated pre-anaesthetic clinics (Armitage, Howat & Long 1974). However, most anaesthetists now recognise that they can safely devolve the selection process to experienced nurses, working within clearly agreed guidelines.

Protocol for determining suitable patient selection

An integrated day unit may experience fewer selection problems than a day ward or surgical ward since experienced staff can more readily implement selection protocols at the pre-assessment interview. They can also consult with clinicians where there may be any doubt.

See Chapter 1

However, although the integrated day unit is the ideal, they are by no means always the norm in district general hospitals. Day case surgery is still performed within day wards, in-patient wards and out-patient clinics. It is therefore going to be difficult for day ward nurses, and probably logistically impossible for the surgical ward nurse, to determine patient suitability before admission.

One solution to this might be to use the expertise of the out-patient nurse. A joint policy written in co-operation with

Box 2.2 Twenty vital questions for safe selection

1. Health status - is the patient physically fit?

2. Does the patient know what operation s/he is to have?

3. How much does the patient know about the day surgery procedure?

4. Has the patient had any previous operation? (day case or in-patient)

5. Has the patient had anaesthetics before? (any reaction or family allergy)

6. Does the patient know what to do about preparing for the operation?

7. Can s/he arrange time off work or help with family commitments?

8. Has the patient suitable surroundings in which to recover?

9. Does the patient have suitable and readily accessible toilet, bathing facilities?

10. Does the patient have transport to and from hospital?

11. Has the patient a suitable and responsible escort and social support?

12. Does the patient know that s/he must have time to recover at home?

13. Does the patient know that s/he must not drive for 48 hours after general anaesthetic?

14. Can the responsible carer get time off work? (?2 days)

15. Is transport or distance from the hospital a problem?

16. Will mobility be impaired? Will s/he need assistance? (i.e. physiotherapy)

17. Can pain be controlled easily at home?

18. Will the patient need assistance from community/practice nurse/GP?

19. Will follow-up or treatment be necessary at the hospital?

20. Does the patient know what to do and who to call if in doubt or in an emergency?

out-patient nurses would provide some guarantee that answers to the questions in Box 2.2 could be communicated, and problems solved, by ward nurses before the patient is admitted. Obviously, for this system to function well, out-patient departments would need to be adequately resourced with trained pre-assessment nurses. They could also become valuable members of the day surgery team since they would be able to assess patients immediately after their out-patient consultation. This would result in considerably less inconvenience to patients as the delay to see the day surgery pre-assessment nurse could be avoided.

Box 2.2 is offered here as the basis for a joint protocol with out-patient nurses. The need for clearly explicit guidelines for day surgery selection and organisation cannot be over-emphasised. Last-minute cancellations are a source of great irritation, inconvenience, stress and anxiety to patients and they are often the result of an inefficient organisation.

See Chapter 3

Because of the need for accurate and effective assessment for day surgery, this important aspect of day surgical nursing is discussed in more depth in Chapter 3.

Protocols for suitable procedures for day surgery

Operational policies should identify which types of surgical procedure are suitable, bearing in mind the length of operating sessions, and the preferences and skills of individual surgeons. No protocols remain static, particularly in day surgery. It will be necessary to revise these regularly as surgical and anaesthetic

Box 2.3   **Some operations suitable for a day surgery unit**

Gynaecological
Laparoscopy
Dilatation and curettage
Excision of cervical lesions
Bartholin cyst excision
Termination of pregnancy
Contraceptive management
Vulval lesions

Oral surgery
Surgical removal of wisdom teeth
Dental clearance
Orthodontic transplant, exposure
Apicectomy
Removal of oral lesions, cysts

Urology
Cystocopy, lesion resection
Urethral stricture, dilatation
Orchidopexy
Excision, marsupialisation of hydrocoele
Circumcision, frenuloplasty
Vasectomy
Congenital herniae

Plastic surgery
Excision of basal cell lesions
Skin grafting
Reduction of prominent ears
Removal of tattoos – birth marks
All minor plastic surgery procedures

Orthopaedic
Arthroscopy – meniscectomy
Removal of internal/external fixators
Osteotomy, removal of exostosis
Arthroplasty, arthrodesis
Fasciotomy, tendon repair

Trigger finger release
Gangliectomy
Carpal tunnel decompression

ENT
Myringotomy
Reduction of nasal fracture
Nasal cautery
Antral washout
Antroscopy
Excision nasal polyp

General surgery
Injection of varicose veins
Herniorrhaphy
Removal of skin lesions
Anal dilatation
Breast biopsy
Gastroscopy
Haemorrhoidectomy
Colonoscopy
Excision, ablation of ingrown toe nails

techniques advance and as more procedures become appropriate for day case treatment.

Although safe selection, in terms of physical suitability, is extremely important, any procedure which is not suitable for day surgery should be avoided. A broad guide (though not a comprehensive list) of suitable operations is given in Box 2.3. Generally, the nurse will be guided in this area by surgeons and anaesthetists but any procedure which carries a high risk of haemorrhage (e.g. tonsillectomy), difficulty in sustaining pain control (some orthopaedic surgery), or the likelihood of prolonged immobility (bilateral hand or foot surgery) might benefit from a longer hospital stay.

Early recommendations from anaesthetists suggested that surgical procedures performed under general anaesthetic should not normally exceed one hour. Nowadays, as day case anaesthesia becomes more sophisticated, there are many combinations of local and general anaesthesia which avoid some of the after-effects traditionally associated with general anaesthesia, such as nausea, vomiting and drowsiness. This policy can therefore sometimes be relaxed, depending on the type of anaesthetic administered.

The development of shorter-acting anaesthetic agents means that a combination of these and the addition of a regional blockade can provide long-acting pain control for a number of day surgery procedures. Some of these procedures, such as herniorrhaphy, were not initially considered suitable because of the inability to control pain, but are now becoming the norm in most Units.

Pre-operative screening protocol

In busy out-patient clinics, surgeons rarely have time to explain to prospective day patients much more than that they will go home the same day, that they must have nothing to eat or drink and sometimes, but not always, that they may be asked to arrange for an escort to drive them home.

As mentioned above, pre-assessment clinics were set up in some places in an attempt to solve the problems of last-minute cancellation caused by patients arriving unfit on the day of surgery. This, however, frequently meant an additional visit to the hospital. Anaesthetists could not guarantee that they would be available to screen a day case immediately following the surgical consultation in the out-patient clinic.

It was not long before it became clear that nurses, with suitable training and skills, could adequately undertake a structured pre-assessment interview with each day patient, with the facilities available for them to contact an anaesthetist for advice if necessary. Then it is only necessary for the surgeon and anaesthetist to check details on the day of surgery to satisfy themselves that there are no problems which have not been addressed by the nursing pre-assessment.

Where waiting lists are overlong, a 're-screening' protocol should be used. The patient should revisit hospital, usually about four weeks prior to the time of surgery for a reassessment. It is advisable also to arrange for a consultation with their surgeon prior to their visit to theatre to talk over any recent developments or changes.

Where a condition has become more complex over time, it may be necessary to err on the side of safety and to arrange for an in-patient operation.

There should be an agreed day surgery policy which states that patients must always be screened for day surgery and, as a minimum, must:

- be accompanied home;

- have responsible assistance at home for 24 to 48 hours;

See
Chapter 3

- conform to explicitly stated standards of physical fitness (see American Society of Anaesthesiologists classification of physical fitness in Chapter 3);

- have prepared for surgery and anaesthesia by fasting for a requisite period of time.

Protocol for providing information to patients and carers about their roles

If patients are insufficiently prepared, or forget what they have been told verbally, then they may have to be rescheduled as in-patients. It is therefore important that all day patients are provided with clear written and verbal instructions. They need to plan ahead to organise their arrangements to fit in with their day surgery in just the same way as in-patients. So information about the part which patients themselves must play in the organisation of their day cases should be clearly and comprehensively explained.

Explaining what to expect is one way in which to alleviate fear of the unknown. The ability to explain and to dispel fears where possible, to talk patients through the process, is probably one of the most important skills of day surgery nursing. For this reason Chapter 5 covers the subject of information and education for day patients in greater depth.

See
Chapter 5

Some people who have experienced more conventional treatment in hospital will need to come to terms with being discharged from hospital on the same day as their surgery. After all, not long ago

Box 2.4 **Pre-operative preparation – what the patient and the carer need to know**

1. Fasting arrangements and preparation for general anaesthetic

2. Estimated length of time in the hospital and timetable of events

3. Estimated time to organise transport to and from hospital

4. The importance of an escort and when to ask them to come

5. Responsible adult assistance overnight and (?) for up to 48 hours

6. Pain control and what to do in an emergency

7. Arrangements to be made for resting, eating, drinking

8. Estimated return to normal activity, driving and work

9. The importance of comfortable clothing

10. What follow-up arrangements will be made and where to get advice after surgery

their doctor would have insisted that a night or two in hospital was necessary.

Box 2.4 may be useful as a framework for more detailed 'local' information protocols. This kind of information can be used as a framework for the interview with the pre-assessment nurse.

The information provided at this interview might also expand on the surgical procedure, which the surgeon may only have had limited time to explain. However, if this is to be part of the assessment interview then clear procedure-specific information should be agreed with each surgeon.

Written information

The benefits of close collaboration with medical colleagues in order to formulate specific written (and verbal) information should not be underestimated. It is obviously important that no conflicting information is given to patients when they have such an important role themselves to play in preparing for surgery and organising their home circumstances.

Those patients who do not have contact with the staff prior to the day of their surgery should receive written information at the appropriate time, with adequate notice for preparation. They should have time to contact the day surgery with any queries and this can obviously save a great deal of time spent in last-minute explanation, rescheduling and anxiety on the day of surgery.

It was, and probably still is, the case that nurses often defuse difficult situations arising from last-minute cancellations and also have to arrange for unplanned admissions overnight. Therefore, to ensure that patients are fully prepared for surgery and are organised to cope with their own recovery, consistent written information must be provided. This should be given to all patients before admission and must cover both general arrangements and procedure-specific instructions.

Scheduling and timing protocols

To run as efficiently as possible, day surgery lists should work almost to split-second timing. Last-minute cancellations and unexpected admissions to hospital not only produce dissatisfied patients, but also result in under-utilisation of lists and personnel. It can be very time-consuming to track down escorts and carers and to arrange a scarce in-patient bed at the last minute.

Forming scheduling protocols will largely depend upon the specific local conditions of each day unit and they are bound to change frequently. They will need to be versatile enough to take account of the mix of surgical specialities and the preferences, speed and expertise of each surgeon and anaesthetist. Timing also needs to take account of the fact that there is more intermediate surgery, for example hernia and varicose vein surgery, being performed as surgeons become more confident with day surgery.

However, some general points may help towards a smooth-running organisation:

- Scheduling the more 'major' cases first on the list (and preferably in the morning) ensures that these cases are fitter for discharge by the end of the day.

- If a day surgery unit is a 'half day' surgery unit (with two lists each day), then it is advisable to run shorter, perhaps local anaesthetic, afternoon lists.

- Although it is not always possible to predict the time each case will take, some estimate can be made by determining each surgeon's and anaesthetist's working practice.

- Day cases only should be scheduled on lists, with no in-patient procedures, or emergencies 'slotted in' (this is difficult in hospitals where no dedicated day case lists are arranged).

- If there are to be mixed in- and out-patient lists, it is advisable for day cases to be treated first. This allows the maximum recovery time, provides valuable time for information giving and adequate pain control and ensures that the necessary discharge criteria are met.

Recovery and pain control protocols

Recovery

Integrated day surgery units will have their own recovery facilities and if nurses rotate through each area of the unit they will become proficient in recovery technique.

Great strides have been made in modern anaesthesia, but patients who are unconscious always require a high level of nursing expertise. This must be no different, or inferior, to a conventional recovery room or critical care area where unconscious patients are nursed. Although a patient may undergo minor surgery under general anaesthetic, a minor operation does not imply a minor general anaesthetic. Patients are either unconscious or they are not.

Most day surgery units will have a primary recovery area where patients recover from general anaesthesia, to a safe level of consciousness, good airway and purposeful movement.

Once recovered (Steward score of 6, see Box 2.5) they will spend a further period of time in a secondary recovery area. Instead of trolleys, recliner chairs in a non-clinical sitting room area might be provided at this stage as they are more comfortable and more conducive to a quicker recovery.

Box 2.5   The Steward recovery score

Consciousness

awake	2
responsive to stimuli	1
not responding	0

Airway

coughing on command or crying	2
maintaining a good airway	1
airway requires maintenance	0

Movement

moving limbs purposefully	2
non-purposeful movement	1
not moving	0

Modified from Steward D.J. (1975) A simplified scoring system for the post-operative recovery room. *Canadian Anaesthesiology Society Journal* **22**; pp. 111–113.

Pain control (box 2.6)

See Further reading at the end of this chapter

Pain control is an important issue in day surgery which cannot be covered in full detail within this handbook. The following basic facts may help to focus any pre-existing knowledge about pain control specifically to the needs of day surgery patients.

- In day surgery, pain control is best addressed before surgery because of the speed of patient throughput.

- A non-steroidal anti-inflammatory analgesic agent may be prescribed as premedication.

Box 2.6   Pain control for day surgery

Pre-operative	Non-steroidal anti-inflammatory preparation – orally or rectally
Intra-operative	Local anaesthetic block Wound infiltration
Post-operative	1. Patient controlled short-acting opioid 2. Simple analgesia combined with non-steroidal anti-inflammatory preparation
Discharge	Simple oral analgesic preparations with clear instructions Sometimes combine with oral non-steroidal anti-inflammatory preparation

- Anaesthetists who are proficient in day case anaesthesia will frequently combine local anaesthetic blocks intra-operatively, reinforced by patient-controlled analgesia, using a short-acting opioid, in the immediate recovery stage.

- Most experienced anaesthetists do not advocate the use of long-acting opioids because their effects may delay discharge.

- Local anaesthetic blocks wear off. This will happen after the patient has been discharged. It will be a considerable source of dissatisfaction to patients to have their pain controlled in hospital only to suffer as soon as they get home!

- Patients must be provided with an adequate supply of simple analgesia so that they may control their own pain. They should be advised to follow the written instructions carefully about when and how often to take them.

- Comprehensive information about pain control must be given to the carer, because of the amnesic effects which general anaesthesia may have on the patient.

Discharge protocols

Many patients expect to feel one hundred percent fit before they go home. Their belief is that they will not be discharged home until they feel well enough to go. It is very important that patients' expectations are realistic in this respect. They must be made fully aware that they require a period of time at home to recover before the effects of their intervention wear off. This is no different from

---

Box 2.7   Framework for a discharge protocol

Stable vital signs when lying down and standing up

Dressing is intact

Little or no blood loss

Alert and orientated

Can tolerate diet and oral fluids

Able to sit/stand/walk/fully mobile within constraints of recent surgery

Has been provided with mobility aid if required

Has passed urine

Cannula/electrodes removed

Letter sent to GP (by hand or fax)

Written discharge and procedure-specific instructions and advice given to patient and escort

Medication and dressings to take home

Follow-up appointment made

Seen by surgeon/consultant

Seen by anaesthetist

Given advice and telephone numbers, information about what to do in an emergency

ACTION GUIDELINES

- identify some of the barriers to effective management and organisation in day surgery

- agree clear workable protocols with the multi-disciplinary team

- co-ordinate the activity of day surgery through a clearly written operational policy

- write clear protocols on:

  - patient selection
  - information
  - procedures suitable for day surgery, scheduling and timing
  - recovery scoring
  - pain control
  - effective discharge criteria

their in-patient counterparts, except that they are able to recover at home rather than in hospital.

Carers must feel comfortable about taking responsibility for the patient and the only way that this can be achieved is by giving them the necessary information to cope. When asked, they sometimes express concern about how to deal with the side-effects of anaesthesia and surgery.

A journey home can be a nightmare when trying to concentrate on the road while at the same time trying to help a nauseated, drowsy or uncomfortable relative or friend. For this reason those who have to travel for more than one hour may not be considered suitable as a day case. On the other hand, with modern anaesthesia and fewer side-effects, this may be considered less important.

Some day surgery facilities may wish to adhere to a protocol which states that patients require a specified period of time before discharge. However, some patients may require less time and some even more. It is probably more appropriate to prepare a mutually agreed 'fitness for discharge' protocol for patients (see Box 2.7). If nurses are willing to take this responsibility and use their skills to assess whether patients meet these rigorous criteria, then a timescale should not be necessary.

Further reading

JONES, A. & McDONNELL, U. (1993) **Managing the Clinical Resource**. Baillière Tindall, London. Introduces the reader to the concept of purchasers and providers (chapter 8) and discusses the management of resources in health care.

OGG, T.W. (1985) **Anaesthesia Rounds – Aspects of Day Surgery and Anaesthesia**. ICI, Macclesfield. Traces the history of day surgery and lists some of the advantages and disadvantages of day surgery. Gives clear direction towards developing a purpose-built day surgery unit.

SMITH, I., Van HEMELRIJCK, J., WHITE, P.F. & SHIVELY, R. (1991) Effects of local anaesthesia on recovery after outpatient arthroscopy. *Anaesthesia Analgesia*, **73**, pp. 536–539. Describes the lasting effect of local infiltration during a day case arthroscopy under general anaesthetic.

RAY, S. (1994) **Anaesthesia and Pain Management for Day Case Surgery - Short Stay Surgery**. UPDATE, June pp. 966–973. A review of the important points to consider in post-operative pain management.

References

ARMITAGE, E.N., HOWAT, J.M. & LONG, F.W. (1974) A day surgery programme for children incorporating an anaesthetic outpatient clinic. *Lancet* **2**, p. 21.

AUDIT COMMISSION (1990) **A Short Cut to Better Services – Day Surgery in England and Wales**. HMSO London.

AUDIT COMMISSION (1992) **All in a Day's Work: An Audit of Day Surgery in England and Wales**. HMSO, London.

DOBSON, R. (1994) Tomorrow's world. *Health Service Journal* Sept. 1994 p. 13

ROYAL COLLEGE OF SURGEONS (1985) **Guidelines for Day Surgery**. Royal College of Surgeons, London.

ROYAL COLLEGE OF SURGEONS (1992) Report of the Working Party on **Guidelines for Day Case Surgery**, Royal College of Surgeons, London.

STEWARD, D.J. (1975) A simplified scoring system for the postoperative recovery room. *Canadian Anaesthesiology Society Journal,* **22,** pp. 111-113.

STEPHENSON, M.E. (1990) Discharge criteria in day surgery: *Journal of Advanced Nursing* **15,** pp. 601-613.

VALUE FOR MONEY UNIT (1991) **Day Surgery – Making it Happen.** NHS Management Executive. HMSO, London.

3

The Assessment Process

Comprehensive day surgery assessment – Patient participation – The benefits of day surgery for specific patient groups – Why a problem-solving approach to assessment is important – A consistent approach to assessment – The patient's progress: the process of assessment – A short analysis of the process of assessment – Physical assessment – Social assessment – Psychological assessment – Conclusion

THIS CHAPTER: Concentrates on the importance of accurate nursing assessment for day surgery. It is based on the belief that there must be a consistent approach to a comprehensive assessment for each patient. A brief analysis of the components of assessment demonstrates the importance of determining the physical, social and psychological needs of patients, however brief their stay in hospital. It advocates the need for a problem-solving approach to assessment and suggests some strategies to streamline the process.

COMPREHENSIVE DAY SURGERY ASSESSMENT

In a high-volume area such as a busy day surgery unit, task assignment and 'conveyor belt' organisation obviously speed up patient throughput. However, a careful balance needs to be struck between efficiency, or 'output' in terms of numbers, and the degree of sensitivity required to assess and address the individual needs of each patient.

Nurses are trained to assess the needs of the individuals in their care. Therefore, delegation of the selection process from clinicians to experienced nurses is becoming the norm in established day surgery units. Evaluation of a nurse-led pre-assessment clinic has demonstrated an improved service to patients and has achieved consistency in the information given to patients (Bottrill 1994).

PATIENT PARTICIPATION

In the early days, there was some concern that day surgery was an abandonment of the unprepared patient into the care of the unskilled (Cassie 1973).

When nurses assess day patients it is important to determine whether they, and their carers, understand the need for and the extent of their involvement in the process. In the past there has been good evidence to suggest that patients were 'de-activated' and 'deskilled' by the power of the medical profession (Zola 1977). Even though there is a greater move towards consumer involvement in health care, there is still a measure of reluctance from some day case patients to take decisions about their health care (Avis 1994).

Safe day surgery demands detailed assessment of suitability. This is not only because there is a need to ensure a suitable operation or to determine the physical suitability of the patient. A number of patients will display insufficient knowledge, or lack the social support necessary to ensure a trouble-free recovery from a day surgery operation. Some patients are neither prepared for, nor fully understand, the need to manage their own post-operative care. In some cases, previous experience may lead them to expect a longer period of care in hospital than day surgery provides. Their perception of adequate care would entail at least one night in hospital to recover.

THE BENEFITS OF DAY SURGERY FOR SPECIFIC PATIENT GROUPS

Day surgery has particular benefits for some groups of patients, even though they were not previously considered suitable.

Healthy children, people with learning disabilities and elderly but fit people can gain the following benefits from day surgery treatment:

- They will be able to recover in familiar surroundings.

- There will be less disruption to normal routine.

- There will be less trauma from a briefer hospital stay in unfamiliar surroundings. Properly prepared, most children, and people with learning difficulties can cope with strange surroundings during the day, but they often find a night away from home very traumatic (Thorne 1991).

- Older people would often prefer to be able maintain their independence. They may more easily become disoriented following anaesthesia in unfamiliar hospital surroundings. This is particularly relevant to ophthalmic surgery and the sight impaired.

The ability to treat these groups of patients as day cases is dependent upon a good assessment of the following:

- that there is adequate social support in place;

- that parents are confident in their ability to cope;

- that full co-operation can be gained from well-informed carers.

A protocol to determine the suitability of patients for day surgery has already been discussed, but it is important to review this frequently as confidence in treating these different groups of patients grows.

See Chapter 2, Box 2.2, for selection protocols

WHY A PROBLEM-SOLVING APPROACH TO ASSESSMENT IS IMPORTANT

Experienced day surgery nurses are well aware of the importance of determining the physical and social suitability of patients for day procedures. However, they also recognise that the psychological impact of an episode in hospital, whatever the treatment or setting, can be of equal significance to patients. They also know that it is necessary for them to identify the problems and needs of day cases in the same depth as for their in-patient counterparts.

When patients are faced with the prospect of an invasive surgical or diagnostic procedure, a pre-assessment interview with a nurse can be used to discuss the nature of their worries, fears and anxieties. An exploration of their problems can reinforce patients' innate coping mechanisms. It will also provide them with enough reassurance and knowledge to allay or dispel some of their uncertainties and fears.

It cannot be assumed that experiences of, and lasting effects from, invasive treatment for day patients will be any less traumatic than they are for in-patients. Time available for contact with patients is inevitably brief in day surgery. It is crucial, therefore, to use the pre-assessment interview in the same way as an admission assessment is conducted for in-patients.

In high volume areas, with large numbers of patients undergoing treatment, some argue that there is no place for a problem-solving approach to care (Henderson 1982). Others contest that these areas are precisely where a logical, organised and problem-solving approach to care is most needed (Walsh 1985). The speed at which patients go through a busy day surgery unit requires precision in organisation and almost split-second timing. Therefore, it follows that time spent identifying problems at the assessment stage can help to avoid poor outcome and potentially serious complications arising.

Even when time is a scarce resource most nurses recognise the value and importance of a comprehensive assessment which can be used for the following:

- to identify problems and to solve or avoid them;
- to determine and address gaps in knowledge;
- to plan for and discuss specific care needs.

A CONSISTENT APPROACH TO ASSESSMENT

Day surgery nurses, in common with all other nurses, will recognise the benefits of adopting a common set of ideals or philosophies to form a framework around which to plan patient care. This should be the starting point for any process of assessment.

A common set of basic assessment criteria, agreed by the whole day surgery team, will generally guarantee the safe and suitable selection of patients for day surgery (see Box 3.1). It could also be adapted and perhaps expanded to suit the local needs of most facilities.

It may be helpful and logical to work through each assessment using the categories below, arranging and structuring the assessment process to ensure a consistent approach which will cover:

- the physical assessment process and the nature and effect of surgical intervention;
- the social assessment and estimate of adequacy of social support;
- the psychological assessment, self-care ability and informational and educational needs.

THE PATIENT'S PROGRESS: THE PROCESS OF ASSESSMENT

The process of preparation for day surgery should begin as early as possible and that contact can be used as a precious opportunity to explore the physical, social, psychological and educational elements which make up the 'whole' patient.

The first visit to a GP with a problem which could suitably be treated as a day case is an opportunity to explore the implications of this form of treatment. To ensure that patients receive accurate and up-to-date information, some day surgery facilities place great emphasis upon liaison with GPs and their teams on a regular basis. They take the view that GPs will only recommend and explain day surgery to patients if they are thoroughly familiar with the criteria for safe selection.

See
Chapter 8

Day surgery and anaesthesia are dynamic fields of medicine, where new techniques result in constantly changing methods of treatment and an ever-increasing variety of procedures. Because of this there needs to be a mechanism for a continuous exchange of information for GPs which is explored in greater depth in Chapter 8.

Possible ways to help familiarise GPs with the day surgery unit could include:

■ information packs and regular newsletters;

■ a promotional video;

■ road shows, social evenings and regular exchange visits.

A prospective day surgery patient will be referred by a GP to an out-patient department and here the consultant will assess the suitability of the patient's condition for a day case.

Where a pre-assessment system is in operation, it will usually be a nurse, working within agreed selection guidelines, who will follow this consultation with a more detailed assessment. The concept of a 'one stop shop', where patients can be seen in the day surgery unit immediately following their out-patient appointment, is ideal and has the added advantage that they can become familiar with the geography of the unit.

Nurse-led pre-assessment, which takes place on the same day as the out-patient consultation, is gradually becoming the norm in many established day surgery units and is generally considered more convenient to patients.

Nurses who conduct pre-assessment interviews need to be adequately trained, and able to seek medical or anaesthetic advice

---

Box 3.1 Suggested list of selection guidelines

- Patients must be accompanied home

- Patients should have inside toilet facilities and a telephone

- The journey home should not exceed one hour

- Patients should be fit and healthy (ASA class 1 or 2, see Box 3.2)

- Avoid operations where severe post-operative pain or haemorrhage may arise

- Exclude all patients who are grossly obese, have imperfectly controlled diabetes mellitus, chronic respiratory or cardiovascular disease

- Laparoscopy patients should weigh less than 80 Kg

- No food or fluids orally for 4 hours prior to general anaesthesia

- Operations should generally not exceed 60 minutes

---

at any time. It is important to lay down rigorous guidelines and to agree on what criteria will support safe selection in consultation with medical colleagues. Once agreed, these selection guidelines must be followed by the whole team. A suggested list of selection guidelines is shown in Box 3.2.

Where patients are seen at outreach clinics, which are often some distance from the day surgery unit, out-patient nurses could take on the assessment of patients. This would avoid the inconvenience of a special pre-assessment visit to the hospital. Familiarity with the selection criteria will mean that both the surgeon and the out-patient nurse can discuss and explore the suitability of day surgery with the patient. Maintaining a regular liaison with these nurses will have the added advantage of fostering good communication, and a supply of questionnaires, written information and instructions can be provided for these clinics.

A SHORT ANALYSIS OF THE PROCESS OF ASSESSMENT

The modern shift towards briefer hospital stays, even for more major procedures, implies the need for a streamlined approach to assessing the suitability and needs of an increasing number of patients.

Consumer-oriented health care and Government charter initiatives suggest that patients should be encouraged to participate more fully in choices and decisions about their own care. There is still evidence that many patients still do not demand a great degree of involvement in decisions about their treatment (Avis 1994).

Most nurses will have encountered a patient who responds passively and predictably in a 'whatever you think best' role. There is obviously a mismatch which needs to be addressed between this philosophy and the concept of patient-centred care. It is important to discuss options and choices at an early stage in the assessment process, to encourage a higher level of patient participation in day surgery.

A multi-factorial, multi-disciplinary approach to the assessment process for day surgery should acknowledge the importance of good patient selection. However, it must be emphasised that selection should not be based on physical suitability alone, but must also acknowledge the importance of psychosocial support. The assessment interview will also offer general guidance to patients, in response to gaps in knowledge, about the treatment proposed and will be supported by procedure-specific, clearly written information which can be read in the less anxiety-provoking atmosphere of home.

PHYSICAL ASSESSMENT

The American Society of Anaesthesiologists (ASA) guidelines set out in Box 3.2 have been advocated as a suitable framework to determine physical suitability for day surgery, in this country and the USA. Because they have been found to work well as simple descriptions of physical criteria, they have been widely adopted,

Box 3.2   **The American Society of Anaesthesiologists' (ASA) classification of physical status**

Class 1
The patients has no organic, physiological, biochemical or psychiatric disturbance. The pathological process for which surgery is to be performed is localised and does not entail a systemic disturbance.

Examples: a fit patient with an inguinal hernia, a fibroid uterus in an otherwise healthy woman.

Class 2
Mild to moderate systemic disturbance caused by either the condition to be treated surgically or by other pathophysiological processes.

Examples: non- or only slightly, limiting organic heart disease, mild diabetes, essential hypertension or anaemia. The extremes of age may be included here, even though no discernible systemic disease is present. Extreme obesity and chronic bronchitis may be included in this category.

Class 3
Severe systemic disturbance or disease from whatever cause, even though it may not be possible to define the degree of disability with finality.

Examples: severely limiting organic heart disease, severe diabetes with vascular complications, moderate to severe degrees of pulmonary insufficiency, angina pectoris or healed myocardial infarction.

Class 4
Severe systemic disorders that are already life threatening, not always correctable by operation.

Examples: patients with organic heart disease showing marked signs of cardiac insufficiency, persistent angina or active myocarditis, advanced degrees of pulmonary, hepatic, renal or endocrine insufficiency.

> **Class 5**
> The moribund patient who has little chance of survival but is submitted to operation in desperation.
>
> Examples: the burst abdominal aneurysm with profound shock, major cerebral trauma with rapidly increasing intracranial pressure, massive pulmonary embolus. Most of these patients require operation as a resuscitative measure with little, if any, anaesthesia.

and adapted for day surgery protocols in this country. As a general rule, most anaesthetists are comfortable with accepting patients for day case general anaesthesia. who conform to class 1 or 2 in the box.

The practice of using a comprehensive health status questionnaire (see Table 3.1), has been adopted in many day surgery units to streamline the assessment process. These questionnaires are designed for completion by the patient, preferably at the assessment interview before admission, when there is still time to address any problems which may need to be solved before admission. The questions asked can form the basic framework for the assessment interview, prompting discussion and information exchange.

Table 3.1 can be used as a basis for physical, social and psychological assessment. The questions are posed so that those who need to read it can identify, at a glance, any potential problems. If any answers are in the 'yes' column, these generally indicate the need for further investigation. (Prompts for the nurse have been added in the last column but do not necessarily need to appear on the patients copy.)

This example can be adapted to suit individual local needs. It has been found to be very useful in busy departments where large volumes of assessment interviews are conducted. A questionnaire published by the Royal College of Surgeons in their **Guidelines for Day Case Surgery** (1992) is also accompanied by a detailed examination of each question to help the assessor to determine

Table 3.1   Health Status Questionnaire

Please ask the patient to complete this. Once completed please discuss with the assessment nurse.

	✓YES	✓NO	Action required if YES
1. Do you have asthma or bronchitis?			Request CXR
2. Have you ever had chest pain or ay other chest problems?			Request ECG and CXR
3. Do you have a cough, cold or nose trouble?			Discuss with anaesthetist
4. Are you breathless on exertion or at night?			Request CXR, Spirometry
5. Do you smoke? (specify how many)?			Discourage prior to anaesthetic
6. Do you drink alcohol, how much each day?			Advise on unit limits, ?LFTs
7. Have you ever had any of the following:			
Heart disease			? Unsuitable for day surgery
Rheumatic fever			ECG
High blood pressure			Check B/P, if ↑ refer to GP
Arthritis			Arthritic neck – refer to anaesthetist
Prolonged muscle weakness			MS Myasthenia – unsuitable
Anaemia			FBC, Hb < 10g – unsuitable
Other blood problems			? Sickle Cell disease – unsuitable
Jaundice			? Hepatitis B screen
Diabetes			? Poorly controlled – unsuitable
Kidney or urinary problems			Urinalysis and U & Es
Sugar in your urine			? Refer to physicians
Swollen ankles			Check B/P, if ↑ refer to GP
Sleeping difficulties			Advise on effect of GA & sedation
Indigestion or heartburn			Refer to anaesthetist
Any other serious illness (if yes please specify)			Refer to anaesthetist
8. Will this be your first operation?			Explain full procedure
9. Will this be your first general anaesthetic?			Explain full procedure
10. If not, did you experience any problems?			Refer to anaesthetist and surgeon
11. Have any of your family had any problems with anaesthetics?			? Malignant Hyperthermia
12. Do you faint easily?			Check B/P, if ↓ refer to GP
13. Do you bruise or bleed a lot?			Clotting screen
14. Are you pregnant?			Unsuitable
15. Do you have any reactions to medicines, tablet or inhalation?			Record all allergies
16. have you eaten or drunk 4/6 hours before your admission?			Complete on admission, if yes CANCEL
17. Will you need any pain killing tablets at home?			Advise on suitable preparation

18. Who will take you home?	23. Do you anticipate any difficulty in coping at home after your operation?
19. Do you have someone to look after you for 24 hours?	24. Do you understand what operation you are having?
20. Do you have private transport home?	25. Do you have any concerns which we should know about?
21. Do you have a telephone?	
22. Do you have access to a lavatory?	

I am aware that if I am having a general anaesthetic/sedation, I know that I must not drive, make any important decisions or operate a cooker or other machinery for at least **24 hours**.
I am aware that I must have a responsible adult with me overnight.

Signature of Patient

the suitability of patients, and the action required, in response to each patient's answer to the questions.

SOCIAL ASSESSMENT

Many prospective day surgery patients expect to leave hospital feeling completely fit. They do not always appreciate the need for an escort home, nor do they expect to have to be cared for once they get home.

When measuring the quality of care in day surgery, the Audit Commission (1991) found that 20% of patients expressed concern about:

- the speed with which they were discharged before they felt fully recovered;

- something going wrong once at home;

- the lack of sufficient rest at home;

- being an extra burden on relatives.

Both the patient and their carer must appreciate that recovery may not be complete for some days, occasionally even a few weeks, depending on the nature of the procedure. If this is not understood then they may feel justifiably aggrieved if their return to normal everyday activities takes longer than they expect.

An assessment of social support should be one of the most strictly enforced criteria when selecting patients for day surgery. All patients must:

- have an escort to get home;

- have suitable private transport;

- have care and support once at home.

Patients must be able to guarantee that they will have sufficient care and support from a responsible, well-informed adult, at least during the first 24 hours at home. A child will not do! As this is a critical safety factor in the recovery process, the assessment should not continue without the guarantee that a carer will be available.

If it is difficult for a patient to find an adult who is willing and able to take on this responsibility, there may need to be some negotiation about suitable dates for treatment. In order to fit in with both patient and carer availability there must be time to arrange convenient time off work.

It is beneficial, but not always possible, to arrange a pre-assessment interview with the patient and their chosen carer. This ensures that both are given the same information, and also the level of knowledge and confidence to take on the responsibility of post-operative care can be assessed.

Additionally, once patients are made aware of the importance of supervision in the post-operative period, they may not always find a day surgery procedure the most convenient option. If there is any doubt about social support then they must be given the option of a night in hospital, or an in-patient procedure, purely on social grounds.

PSYCHOLOGICAL ASSESSMENT

Determining the impact of day surgery upon the perceptions and emotions of each patient is probably just as important as gauging the less abstract physical and social components of assessment. Because this will obviously require an adequate amount of time, it should not be left to the day of admission and must form part of the pre-assessment interview.

It is important that the nurse assessing the day patient is skilled enough to recognise and to note the attitude of each day patient towards their treatment. Responses to the following questions can be noted in the form of a brief narrative, forming part of the assessment questionnaire:

- Will this be your first operation?
- Do you understand what operation you are having?
- Will this be your first general anaesthetic?
- Do you anticipate any difficulty in coping at home after your operation?
- Do you have any concerns that we should know about?

See Further reading

Health professionals do not always appreciate that day surgery can have the same impact on the anxiety levels of patients as a more major procedure. (Some suggestions for further reading on this subject is at the end of this chapter.)

Those patients who display high levels of anxiety, and whose previous experience has influenced their view of surgery may benefit from in-patient care rather than the brief period of contact with health professionals which day surgery implies. It should therefore be open to all patients to decline a day surgical procedure if they feel that they could not cope with their own post-operative care.

See Chapter 4 where a framework for nusing in day surgery is discussed

The future direction for nursing must lie in supporting the self-care ability of a more knowledgeable public as day surgery increases and shorter hospital visits become the norm. The underlying theory of self-care will be given more attention in Chapter 4.

See Chapter 5 for education, information and patient teaching

It is important to emphasise in any brief discussion on the psychological aspects of nursing care that the past experiences of patients, whether gained personally or vicariously, are bound to have an effect, adverse or otherwise, on their perceptions and attitudes. It is important, then, to spend time during the assessment process in determining what these perceptions and attitudes are. Only then can a plan be formulated which will educate and inform patients about the implications, as they perceive them, of their hospital visit. This extremely important aspect of day surgery is covered in more detail in Chapter 5.

CONCLUSION

When assessing patients for day surgery, it is important not to lose sight of the fact that the philosophy of day surgery nursing has to be largely one of support for patients during what is often an enforced period of self-care until they are fit to resume their normal life.

It will, therefore, be the responsibility of the nurses in day surgery to use their powers of assessment to ensure that each patient's ability for self-care is not compromised, and that each patient has

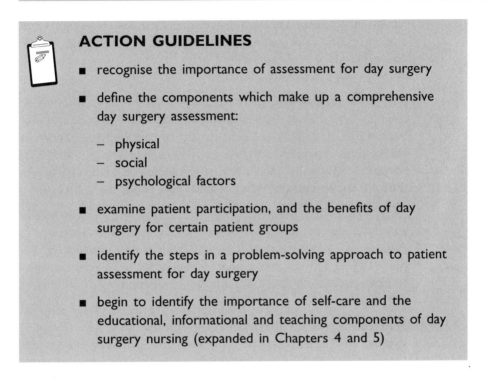

ACTION GUIDELINES

■ recognise the importance of assessment for day surgery

■ define the components which make up a comprehensive day surgery assessment:

– physical
– social
– psychological factors

■ examine patient participation, and the benefits of day surgery for certain patient groups

■ identify the steps in a problem-solving approach to patient assessment for day surgery

■ begin to identify the importance of self-care and the educational, informational and teaching components of day surgery nursing (expanded in Chapters 4 and 5)

the knowledge, social support and psychological frame of mind to cope during the recovery period at home.

Since the expansion of day surgery, there has been considerable debate on the subject of pre-operative selection, generally focusing on the physical criteria for patient suitability. This chapter has attempted to identify the special skills which nurses can bring to the selection process. They are concerned not only with physical aspects of assessment, but also with the social and psychological functioning of patients. Safe selection can only be guaranteed, therefore, by a detailed and comprehensive, multi-faceted assessment process.

People are being urged to demand more knowledge about themselves and their treatments. This challenges the traditional function of nursing by shifting the emphasis from physical 'hands on' care, towards a psychological, supportive and educative role. In day surgery this implies the need to develop finely tuned communication skills to convey information in a shorter period of time and in difficult circumstances. Achieving this will enhance the image and credibility of day surgery nursing in the eyes of both public and professional colleagues.

Further reading

BANDURA, A. (1977) Self-efficacy: towards a unifying theory of behavioural change. *Psychological Review* **84**, pp. 191–215. Suggested that some psychological strategies can help to control a health care situation.

GIDRO-FRANK, L., GORDON, T. & TAYLOR, H.L. (1988) Pelvic pain and female identity: a survey of emotional factors in forty patients. *American Journal of Obstetrics and Gynaecology* **79**, pp. 1183–1203. Suggests that assessment of personality characteristics can be reliable as predictors of outcome.

NICHOLS, K.A. (1984) **Psychological Care in Physical Illness**. Beckenham, Croom Helm. Discusses the need for psychological support and the importance of patient participation in health care.

ROTTER, J.B. (1954) **Social Learning and Clinical Psychology**. Prentice Hall, Englewood Cliffs, NJ. Describes the assumptions that people perceive either an external or internal cause for their present predicament and perception of their own self-efficacy, capabilities and levels of motivation.

SCHLOESSLER, M. (1989) Perceptions of pre-operative education in patients admitted the morning of surgery: *Patient Education and Counselling,* **14**, pp. 127–136 Examines the anxiety-provoking nature of diagnostic minor surgery.

References

AMERICAN SOCIETY OF ANAESTHESIOLOGISTS (1963) New classification of physical status. *Anaesthesiology* **24**, p. 111.

AUDIT COMMISSION (1991) **Measuring Quality: The Patient's View of Day Surgery**. HMSO, London.

AVIS, M. (1994) Choice cuts: an exploratory study of patients' views about participation in decision-making in a day surgery unit. *International Journal of Nursing Studies 31* **3**, pp. 289–298.

BOTTRILL, P. (1994) Nursing assessment prior to day surgery. *The Journal of One Day Surgery* **4–2**, p. 23.

CASSIE, A.(1973) Surgery in day patients. *British Medical Journal* **1** p. 542.

HENDERSON, V. (1982) The nursing process - is the title right?' *Journal of Advanced Nursing* **7**, pp. 103-109.

ROYAL COLLEGE OF SURGEONS (1992) **Guidelines for Day Case Surgery**, 2nd edn. Royal College of Surgeon of England, London.

THORNE, R. (1991) **Just for the Day – Caring for Children in the Health Service**. NAWCH, London.

WALSH, M. (1985) **Accident and Emergency Nursing: A New Approach**. Heinemann, London.

ZOLA, I.K. (1977) Health and disabling medicalization. **Disabling Professions**. Marion Boyars, New York.

4
A Nursing Framework for Day Surgery

The need for a framework for day surgery nursing –
Some common characteristics of the day surgery patient
– A philosophy for nursing in day surgery – Self-care –
A practical application for nursing theory – Care mapping
– A short case history – Conclusion

THIS CHAPTER: Describes the use of a nursing plan to streamline the process of day surgery based on some common characteristics identified in day surgery patients. It recommends the use of a common philosophy for nursing in day surgery. It examines the theory of self care as a suitable framework for day surgery nursing and uses this theoretical framework to suggest a practical and workable mapping process, with a suggested example. The main aim of this chapter is to identify strategies which may help to provide an effective and consistent nursing service for day surgery patients.

THE NEED FOR A FRAMEWORK FOR DAY SURGERY NURSING

Having emphasised the importance of accurate assessment and rigorous selection for day surgery in Chapter 3, this chapter takes the process a step further. A framework is suggested to support the nursing process of assessment, planning, intervention and evaluation. Any nursing process will, however, only work if it consists of practical steps which realise the ultimate goal of day surgery – that of ensuring the process of care is a reliable, consistent and high quality experience for all patients.

Even the most effective assessment and selection process cannot always guarantee that every patient arrives for day surgery without any problems. There will always be some misconceptions and misunderstandings, which inevitably take time to resolve.

See
Chapter 3

However, most day patients will share some similar attributes because they will have been assessed as conforming to the selection guidelines discussed in Chapter 3. Because of these shared characteristics many interventions will be similar and therefore a basic plan can be prepared for many patients. This will release valuable time to address those factors which are individual or unique to each patient.

The maintenance of accurate written records of nursing care can also be addressed by providing a versatile core document. All these plans must provide additional space for noting individual needs or problems once they have been identified.

SOME COMMON CHARACTERISTICS OF THE DAY SURGERY PATIENT

A consistent approach to nursing care starts, then, by building a framework based on the following common characteristics shared by most day surgery patients. These are that:

- they are usually relatively fit and healthy;

- they are generally, but not always, within an age group where there is a strong probability of suitable social support;

- they will not be undergoing a procedure that requires intensive post-operative support or critical care;

- most 'self-care deficits' experienced by day patients lie in lack of education, inadequate understanding or knowledge to deal with what does happen to them;

■ they often fail to appreciate the importance of their part in the proceedings.

If it can be assumed that most patients share these characteristics, then individual problems will stand out and be identified more easily. Some of these problems will already have been addressed at pre-assessment as a result of responses to the self-assessment health status questionnaire.

See Chapter 3

A PHILOSOPHY FOR NURSING IN DAY SURGERY

A number of task-based nursing interventions can be performed efficiently and relatively effectively by teaching basic skills and these can be easily measured. However, the care of the *whole* person is altogether more complicated and implies a need to 'flesh out' those basic skills, guided by thought and reflection. This can be done by agreeing a precise set of commonly held beliefs about the nature of day surgery nursing and by recognising that, even though they may share some common characteristics, all day surgery patients have individual and specific needs.

Building a philosophical framework within which to care holistically for day surgery patients will obviously require more than merely the acquisition of the technical abilities needed for perioperative nursing care. A philosophy will, after all, vary according to the unique needs of patients in every setting where nursing takes place.

One of a number of dictionary definitions for the word 'philosophy' describes it as a particular system and set of beliefs which is reached through seeking truth, understanding and gaining knowledge about reality.

The acquisition of a nursing philosophy, therefore, implies that there is a need to pursue and discover truths about human behaviour in health and illness in order to understand it. A philosophical approach can also contribute to a much wider understanding of the whole person requiring care, and should form part of a basic framework within which to build upon the patient/nurse relationship.

Box 4.1   **Building a philosophy of nursing care for day surgery**

1. The aims of nursing
We aim to care for our patients by recognising that each is an individual, requiring support and expertise during their short time with us.

We aim to provide cost-effective and efficient care, while recognising that our patients are active participants in their own care.

2. The concept which underpins nursing care
We place emphasis upon the concept of self-care; in that each person is required to arrive prepared for their operation and will re-assume responsibility for their own care when discharged home.

3. The role of the nurse
The role of the nurse is primarily that of a supporter and educator, who, nevertheless, is required to be skilled in all aspects of surgical nursing care, operative technique and recovery room skills.

4. The rationale of care
Given the compressed time-frame available for nursing care, technical proficiency, assessment, judgment and organisational skills must be highly refined. Flexibility will allow nurses in the unit to function in all areas of the facility.

5. The special nature of day surgery patients
The nurse in the day surgery unit will recognise that to each of her patients their operation is a major source of anxiety and will be a stressful event, however minor their condition may seem. Also, for those undergoing a general anaesthetic, there is no such thing as a 'minor' general anaesthetic. Therefore, the nurse is required to act for patients during this time, but is able to relinquish care to them by ensuring that they have enough information to resume their own care when discharged home.

> **6. The patient-centred focus**
> The day surgery unit is the ideal place to observe the total
> nursing process within a short period of time. It must,
> however, be recognised that it has been conceived as a
> service to patients, so that they do not have to wait too
> long for their operations. They have the right to expect a
> service carried out by a dedicated multidisciplinary team
> whose experienced practice is focused upon safe, efficient
> and cost-effective care.

Box 4.1 provides a set of philosophical beliefs which could be
adapted for individual use. It has been devised to reflect the self-
caring nature of the day patient and defines the position of nursing
in day surgery. It can be adapted to build an explicit philosophy
for nursing day surgery patients in individual units.

Because of the 'common characteristics' that have already been
identified, day surgery nurses will usually be able to predict that
their contribution to care lies in assuming a supportive, guiding
and educative role for a (normally) self-caring individual.
Therefore, as each person goes through the unfamiliar process of
day surgery they will require varying levels of nursing support,
education and information to reinforce their innate ability for
self-care.

SELF-CARE

There is very little time to get to know a patient well in day
surgery units. However, it is necessary to assess self-care ability,
since it cannot be assumed that patients will be able to co-operate
in their own care.

No nursing theorist advocates a total take-over of the conscious
patient without first seeking their input into the planning of
their care and their co-operation in the setting of goals and
achieving agreed outcomes. In the past, however, these views
have been contrary to the philosophy of some medical and nursing
professionals, who have subscribed to the view that they know

what is best for their patients. They have been used to taking decisions on behalf of, and without reference to, their patients. Also, many patients have accepted this situation by acknowledging that 'doctor knows best'. These people would prefer to leave their care to the 'experts'. But such philosophies and attitudes are gradually changing. People are beginning to demand a greater say in what happens to them when they need hospital treatment.

It is true to say that patients are not always given total freedom to choose whether they would prefer a day case or an in-patient stay. They are often confronted with longer delays if they opt for an in-patient procedure and therefore choose day surgery only because they will be treated more quickly. Therefore, when assessing patients for day surgery, it is important to remember that many of them will need support in what can be an unfamiliar and anxiety-provoking self-caring role.

More explanation of 'self-care', as defined by Orem (1985), is appropriate here. Most of the 'theoretical' principles of the self-care model can be readily applied to day patients (see text in italics).

The basic beliefs underlying this theory are as follows:

- People are self-caring and only require nursing if they have self-care limitations – *Day patients are expected to be self-caring both before and after their surgery.*

- Health is described as 'soundness', and physical and mental well-being – *During the day surgery procedure, nursing must provide the support, guidance and care to compensate for health deficits brought about through the effects of anaesthesia, anxiety and surgical intervention.*

- Nursing systems provide nursing to regulate a person's self-care abilities – *The role of the day surgery nurse is to assist in assessing suitability and to rectify deficits in self-care ability.*

- Nursing will provide an environment which is conducive to development and growth – *The day patient needs to assimilate enough knowledge to make suitable arrangements to control their own environment themselves, both before and after their hospital treatment.*

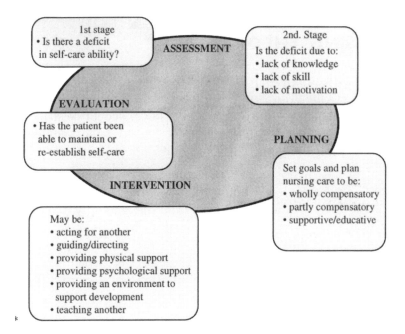

Fig. 4.1   Diagrammatic map of self-care theory, from Orem (1985).

This brief analysis of the self-care model demonstrates that, perhaps without being fully aware of it, most nurses who care for short-stay hospital patients subscribe to the concept of 'self-care'. They expect their patients to 'prepare' and 'care' for themselves within their own environment. Thus, both pre- and post-operative care shifts away from the nurse and onto the patient. It follows, too, that nursing expertise will only need to be mobilised at those times when an individual does not have the capacity to maintain his own self-care.

Figure 4.1 is a visualisation of the theory of self-care. It unites the familiar steps of the nursing process to Orem's identification of 'deficits' in a patient's self-care ability. It categorises the nature of nursing intervention required and caters for an evaluation of return to self-care ability, or otherwise (when the process may need to be repeated), at the end of an episode of care.

A PRACTICAL APPLICATION FOR NURSING THEORY

Any attempt to apply 'pure' nursing theory to everyday nursing practice is difficult in any field of nursing. However, because of very brief contact with patients, every effort should be made to streamline nursing care plans to cater for the large number of patients going through day surgery units.

Many nursing theorists could be regarded purely as 'thinkers', and their considerable contribution to the profession will only be useful if their ideas are translatable from the 'know that' into the practical 'know how' of day-to-day nursing care (Field 1987). Also, many theories have been devised with the purpose of making explicit a common purpose (or philosophy) on which to build and plan consistent standards of care. Therefore:

- Theory will only be useful if it is relevant to every day practice.

- Theory should be examined in depth if it is to be used to formulate philosophy and standards.

See Further
reading at
the end of
this chapter

- Theory should be clear to everyone if it is to become an implicit framework around which every nurse is expected to plan and evaluate care (some further reading may help).

- If theory becomes an integral part of nursing practice, it will remove the need for lengthy, explicit instructions and prescriptive procedural explanations.

It is not, however, the purpose of this handbook to do more than draw out a few components from a range of theories where they may be useful to illustrate or clarify the special needs of day patients. Figure 4.2 sets out a few of the basic philosophies from Orem and other theorists as they may relate to nursing care in day surgery. It demonstrates the way in which theories can be incorporated into an eclectic approach when formulating a philosophy for day surgery patients.

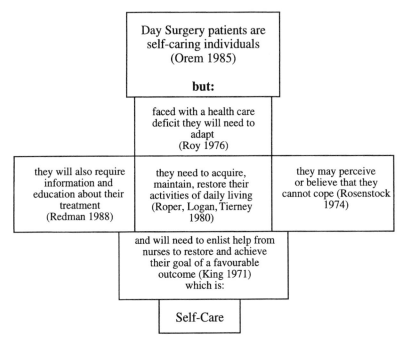

Fig. 4.2   Some theories which underpin a day surgery care-plan.

CARE MAPPING

Theories can be important as building blocks or support towards effective nursing practice. Practice must also be underpinned by practical systems of delivering and documenting care provided. Most nurses would agree that close contact with patients and meaningful 'bedside' nursing can be only too easily compromised by the need to document all care provided. This is obviously a particular problem in high volume areas such as day surgery.

In the day surgery setting, then, there needs to be an efficient method of documenting the care process and a care map is just such a system. A care map is an efficient and comprehensive solution. It can provide a framework, linked to expected outcomes, for planning and ensuring appropriate delivery of care within set time periods. It can also be used for concurrent and retrospective audit from variations in the expected progress of patients (Hale & Laxade 1995).

The speed of throughput suggests that pro-active management of care through mapping the predicted progress of patients may be an option which could help to solve this. Additions to a care map will only need to be made where variations (variances) to predicted progress occur. These maps should be designed with input from all the staff. They are particularly effective if they can be interdisciplinary, and they can save valuable time. Time-saving strategies mean that nurses will be able to use the time saved for more patient contact, education and support.

Care maps must, however, meet the following criteria if they are to be effective:

■ They should cover the whole process of care through the day surgery system.

■ They should be familiar and 'user friendly' to everyone, including patients.

■ They must be versatile enough to chart variations from the 'normal' path. A map will show the required predictable interventions, with scope to document those areas which are unique to each patient.

See
Chapter 5
for more
detail

■ They must be accompanied by consistent information to prevent ambiguous messages being transmitted.

■ They should demonstrate that less time is wasted as each patient is 'mapped' through the process. The nurse will be released from excessive documentation to provide vital individual support, guidance and education to patients.

■ They must be able to be easily audited. Interventions must be evaluated in terms of outcomes for each patient. They can be used to audit the incidence of unresolved problems which may have led to diversion or cancellation of treatment from day surgery (variance analysis).

A SHORT CASE HISTORY

Using the care map illustrated in Table 4.1 it should be possible to incorporate Orem's nursing systems into a map of the care suitable for most day case patients. 'There is evidence that most patients with a particular condition have, despite their individuality, a set of generic problems and need similar interventions to meet the desired . . . outcomes' (Zander 1992).

The basic nursing philosophy of self-caring patients, only requiring the assistance from experts when their self-care abilities are compromised through illness, lack of knowledge or skill, can be demonstrated by the following short case history.

Since her gynaecologist had judged her suitable for day surgery, Susan arrived at the day surgery unit straight from her appointment at the gynaecological clinic to arrange for a diagnostic laparoscopy for the following week. Her history of primary infertility suggested that this was to be a diagnostic procedure to determine the cause.

*Her health status questionnaire was completed and this confirmed that her general health was good, although she had never had a general anaesthetic or operation before. There was no **physical** deficit identified which would indicate that a day surgery procedure would be unsafe but there were some knowledge deficits to be addressed.*

Assessment

First stage   Second stage

Is there a deficit in self-care ability because of physical, social or psychological factors?

Is the deficit due to:
■ **lack of skill**
■ **lack of knowledge**
■ **lack of motivation?**

*Susan did, however, demonstrate from her completion of the questionnaire, and in discussion with the day surgery nurse, that she had some **knowledge** deficits about the nature of a general anaesthetic and surgery and the effect it might have on her.*

■ *She was intending to take only one day off work and was unaware that she might need longer at home to recover.*

Table 4.1 Care map for minor surgery

Patient Susan   Operation proposed   Date

Out-patient dept.	Pre-assessment in day surgery	Pre-operative care	Operation	Recovery
Consultation	Assessment by nurse for day case suitability	Role explanation of: named nurse, surgeon, anaesthetist	Informed consent	Conscious levels
Selection assessment	Health status	Fasting/prepared		Vital signs
?Pre-op tests	Knowledge Perceptions	Observations	Safe operative environment	Wound care
Information	Social support available	Height/weight Transport	Act for patient under anaesthetic	Guide, support during recovery
Consent to operation and anaesthetic	Written information	Escort		
	Procedure specific instructions			
	Contact number given	Theatre checklist		
Sig.	Sig.	Sig.	Sig.	Sig.

Sign off each column above as interventions are completed

Table 4.1 (cont.)

Out-patient dept.	Pre-assessment in day surgery	Pre-operative care	Operation	Recovery
Nursing interventions				
Assessment of: physical status psychological status social needs	Deficit in: knowledge skill motivation	Supportive Educative Guide/direct	Wholly compensatory care Create a suitable environment Act for patient	Wholly compensatory care Create a suitable environment Act for patient
VARIANCES/OUTCOME				
EVALUATION				

■ *Because she had been told that she would be well enough to go home the same day as her operation she said that she expected that she would feel completely fit to go home.*

■ *She was not sure that her husband would be able to collect her.*

Planning and intervention

Set goals and plan nursing care to be:	Intervention here is:
1. supportive/**educative**	**guiding/psychological**
2. partly compensatory	**support/teaching/**
3. wholly compensatory	**educating**

A discussion with the day surgery screening nurse emphasised that she would not feel 'back to normal' on discharge home and, therefore, the importance of the support and help she would need, both to get home and at home, was explained. It was clearly demonstrated that, never having experienced surgery or a general anaesthetic before, her reaction and physical condition post-operatively could not be fully predicted. Hence the need to emphasise the importance of forward planning to arrange support from a responsible adult for at least 24 hours afterwards.

Susan was a dental nurse and was obviously familiar with some aspects of the effects of anaesthesia and surgery. Because she had some knowledge, and following a discussion about how she felt about her part in a day surgery operation, she could be considered as psychologically able to cope at home.

It was still important to explain the nature of the procedure, the routine on the day of surgery and her part in preparing for her operation. Together with this verbal information, written information about post-operative limitations, possible symptoms, follow-up arrangements and methods of pain control was also supplied for her to take home and read at leisure.

This information, provided well before the day of surgery, was designed to instil confidence in Susan's ability for self-care. It would ensure that she was able to arrive on the day

of surgery fully prepared and well enough informed to prevent the unpleasant surprises which are often an unwelcome feature of invasive procedures.

Admission

Set goals and plan nursing care to be:
1. supportive/educative
2. **partly compensatory**

3. wholly compensatory

Intervention here is:

guiding/directing/ creating a suitable environment for care

Susan arrived for her surgery, naturally anxious, but well prepared. Post-operative pain control was explained and she was shown how to use a hand-held device with which she could control her own pain. She was seen by her surgeon and anaesthetist and consented to her operation. The same nurse who had assessed her was able to support and guide her throughout the procedure. Other staff had ensured that everything had been prepared in advance for a smooth anaesthetic and trouble-free operation.

Operation and recovery

Set goals and plan nursing care to be:
1. supportive/educative
2. partly compensatory
3. **wholly compensatory**

acting for another/ creating an environment to support care

During the operation and the initial recovery phase Susan's total care was delivered by nurses who were expert in theatre technique and recovery skills. They would act for Susan in the event of any complication arising and they would take responsibility for the safety of the environment in which Susan was placed. By acting for Susan when she was unable to care for herself, they were also prepared for any emergency which is concomitant with anaesthesia and surgical intervention.

Post-operative care

Set goals and plan nursing care to be:	Intervention here is:
1. supportive/educative	providing psychological support/teaching/educating
2. partly compensatory	providing physical support/guiding/directing
3. wholly compensatory	

As soon as Susan was awake she was able to take some responsibility for her own care. For instance, she was encouraged to use her pain-control button which would deliver small doses of a short-acting analgesic whenever she needed it. It is important that every moment in day surgery should be utilised fully. The recovery phase was used to educate and inform Susan about her symptoms, wound care and pain control. It was understood, though, that much of what was said would not be fully assimilated while Susan was still influenced by the amnesic effect of her general anaesthetic. Psychological support from her nurse and a restful environment allowed Susan to restore her own self-care ability.

Within 3 hours Susan was well enough to go home in the care of her husband. Her surgeon took care to explain his operative findings while her husband was present and discussed her future management and aftercare with them both.

Evaluation

Care could not be considered complete until Susan was restored to her own self-caring status and returned to her normal activities of daily living.

This evaluation took the form of a phone call to Susan the following day. This phone call was used to ask a number of questions evaluating her progress towards self-care.

This evaluation concluded that Susan was feeling really well after 24 hours at home. She had taken some of her oral analgesia but had not experienced any severe or referred pain as a result of her laparoscopy.

Her husband had remained at home the day after her operation but she was beginning to get back to normal and was not dependent upon him. She was hoping to return to work the next day and knew that she would be receiving an outpatient appointment to discuss her further management with her gynaecologist.

Susan thought that her care contained all the elements of care which any patient undergoing conventional surgery would expect and did not feel disadvantaged by being a day case. She said that she was given enough information to take over her own care and it could be concluded that the outcome of her care was satisfactory. She was aware that she was going to require further treatment as a result of the findings from her operation and she said that she would have no concerns about having further treatment as a day case.

Box 4.2 is a short questionnaire which can be used as a telephone evaluation for patients. The care map should be signed off only after it has been established, from asking these questions, whether recovery has been uneventful or not.

It is important to determine whether day surgery had been the right course of action for all patients. Day surgery was a success for Susan but some patients will express concern about their recovery process. Understanding the nature of their anxieties will improve and refine the provision of information and support for other patients going through the system.

CONCLUSION

Predetermining those factors which are common to all patients and supporting and guiding patients until they are able to restore their self-care ability has two advantages. It creates more time for

Box 4.2　**Evaluation of progress by telephone after 24 hours**

Some questions to ask:

- How are you feeling?

- How did you feel on your journey home?

- Have you experienced any pain since you got home?

- Have you taken any painkillers, did they work?

- Have you felt dizzy, sick or faint?

- Have you any problems with your wound?

- Did you have to call your GP or community nurse?

- Are you clear about your follow-up or further treatment arrangements?

- Have you any worries we can help you with?

- Did you receive enough information from us?

- Is there anything else you would like to know?

- Do you have any suggestions for improving care if you have to come to hospital as a day patient again?

- Would you recommend this form of treatment to a friend?

significant patient contact while addressing the unique needs or attributes which make each patient an individual.

The simple case history in this chapter highlights a patient's specific needs as she progresses through the day surgery process, and the varying interventions required from the day surgery nurse. The practicalities of documenting a care map specifically for day surgery patients demonstrates that a 'system' can be designed to provide a framework around which to plan, implement and evaluate each specific intervention within a day surgery unit.

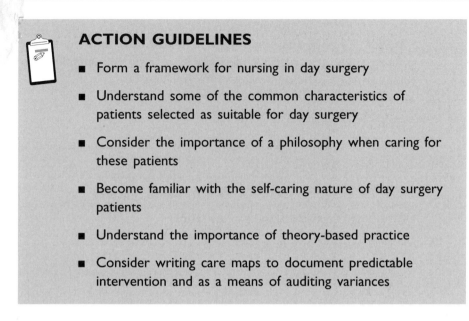

ACTION GUIDELINES

- Form a framework for nursing in day surgery

- Understand some of the common characteristics of patients selected as suitable for day surgery

- Consider the importance of a philosophy when caring for these patients

- Become familiar with the self-caring nature of day surgery patients

- Understand the importance of theory-based practice

- Consider writing care maps to document predictable intervention and as a means of auditing variances

Further reading

KING, I.M. (1971) **Towards a Theory for Nursing**. John Wiley, New York. **Goal and outcome theory**: the nurse and the patient meet in a health care setting and agree to act, react, interact, and transact (or negotiate) to achieve common goals and to reach a successful outcome.

REDMAN, B.K. (1988) **The Process of Patient Education**. C.V. Mosby, St. Louis. **Education theory**: An interpersonal relationship between the nurse, who has knowledge, information and skill and the patient who needs knowledge, information and skill.

ROPER, N., LOGAN, W. & TIERNEY, A. (1980) **The Elements of Nursing**. Churchill Livingstone, Edinburgh. **Activities for daily living**: The nurse assists an individual in acquiring, maintaining or restoring maximum independence in their activities of living.

ROSENSTOCK, I.M. (1974) Historical origins of the health belief model. *Health Education Monographs* 2, pp. 324-508. **Health belief**: The views of an individual; attitudes and beliefs about the perceived severity of their illness, their vulnerability and what action they may take, faced with the threat of illness.

ROY, C. (1976) **Introduction to Nursing: An Adaptation Model**. Prentice Hall, New Jersey. **Adaptation to illness**: The nurse promotes adaptive responses to stressful situations by supporting a patient's own coping mechanisms.

References

FIELD, P.A. (1987) The impact of nursing theory on the clinical decision-making process. *Journal of Advanced Nursing*, **12** pp. 563–571.

LAXADE, S. & HALE, C. (1995) Managed care 1: an opportunity for nursing. *British Journal of Nursing* **4** No.5, pp. 290–294.

OREM, D.E. (1985) **Nursing – Concepts of Practice**. McGraw Hill, New York.

ZANDER, K. (1992) Critical pathways in total quality management. In **The Health Care Pioneers** (eds Melum, M.M. & Sinior, M.K.), pp. 305–314. American Hospital Publishing, Chicago.

5

Patient Information

Introduction – Some general problems and solutions in
information exchange – A well-informed patient minimises
the risks – The nurse's role in providing information –
Conformity and consistency of information – Patients'
rights – Communication skills for effective information
exchange – The balance between written and verbal
information – Conclusion

THIS CHAPTER: Identifies the important part which
nurses must play in providing information and patient
teaching. It offers some basic guidance towards achieving
competence and skill in these important areas. It recognises
the barriers, risks and problems which militate against
successful absorption of facts. It suggests how to minimise a
few of the more major and some of the frequently occurring problems when trying to convey the maximum amount
of information in the shortest possible time.

INTRODUCTION

The needs of day patients differ from those of in-patients in
many ways, most importantly in that they must have sufficient
information to be able to manage their own preparation for
surgery. They must also be given the confidence, through greater
knowledge, to manage their own post-operative recovery when
they leave hospital.

Information in day surgery is crucially important to patients who,
perhaps, will have no-one to reassure them and who must, very

quickly, acquire enough knowledge to manage their own pre- and post-operative care. In the short time which these patients spend in hospital, every contact between a patient and health professional should be used as an opportunity for receiving and giving information.

Before the benefits of a pre-assessment system for day surgery became the norm, it was a source of some concern that a significant number of inadequately prepared patients arrived on the day of surgery displaying very little knowledge about their part in the procedure. A great deal of time needed to be spent, at a time when anxious pre-operative patients had difficulty in absorbing facts, trying to identify suitable escorts and making hurried, last-minute arrangements to ensure a safe discharge.

Therefore, at an early stage in the development of day surgery, it was acknowledged that the quality of information given to patients and their carers had a direct effect upon their acceptance of and satisfaction with the whole process (Garraway *et al.* 1978).

SOME GENERAL PROBLEMS AND SOLUTIONS IN INFORMATION EXCHANGE

If a patient cannot meet the selection criteria they should not be considered suitable candidates for day surgery. Determining knowledge deficit as early as possible provides the screening nurse with time to explain the importance of the patient's own part in the process. Some knowledge deficits can only be rectified before the date of admission and this reinforces the crucial importance of the screening process to ensure safe selection of day cases.

In a day surgery setting, it could be assumed that lack of time makes it too difficult, or even impossible, to address information issues adequately. There are some basic strategies, however, which may help to ensure that patients absorb the important information necessary to cope confidently with their own care:

The problem	A solution
■ Effective and successful exchange of information will become more difficult, if not impossible, if it is delivered while the patient progresses through a day surgery procedure.	■ Information and education must take place before the day on which surgery takes place to allow a patient time to absorb the facts.
■ It is not easy for a patient to assimilate complex terminology and detailed information, offered at a time when anxiety and unfamiliarity militate against successful absorption of facts.	■ Clearly written and verbal information must be available to allow time for patients to ask for clarification.
■ The 'minor' nature of a day surgery procedure may not seem to be a priority, in terms of valuable out-patient time, to a busy surgeon when more 'serious' cases must take precedence.	■ Nurses can use the pre-assessment interview, after an out-patient appointment, to put the procedure into context and can expand on what the patient will experience.
■ It is evident that many patients still do not either receive, or assimilate, enough information during an out-patient appointment.	■ Patients have individual and unique educational needs and nurses can help by translating and interpreting complex information for them.
■ Many of the complaints which health care organisations receive can be directly attributable to inadequate, ambiguous or unintelligible information.	■ The Health Commissioner's reports (Ombudsman) can help to highlight areas of concern and the need for greater clarity in providing information throughout the health service.

> ## Box 5.1   Minimising the risks
>
> Patients are suitable for day surgery only after ensuring that they, and their carers, can:
>
> - be assessed for their ability to grasp the significant differences between this method of surgery and that of in-patient care
>
> - explore the advantages and disadvantages of day surgery to make informed decisions about making alternative arrangements for a conventional in-patient admission in good time
>
> - understand the importance of fasting before anaesthesia and the consequences of not doing so and be aware of the 'normal' side-effects of anaesthesia
>
> - arrange for a responsible escort and understand the reason why they must be driven home and looked after for 24 to 48 hours at home
>
> - be prepared and able to reorganise their lives and the lives of their escorts and carers in order to take time to recover after their treatment

A WELL-INFORMED PATIENT MINIMISES THE RISK

Many day surgery patients do not fully appreciate the nature of their treatment, nor do they always expect to experience adverse symptoms once they have left hospital. Therefore, minimising the risk associated with poorly informed day surgery patients is only possible if, following information exchange, they are able to demonstrate a full and comprehensive understanding of the implications of all stages of their treatment and recovery period.

See Chapter 3 where assessment is covered in more detail

The assessment interview must include a comprehensive assessment of the patient's ability to assimilate information. This must obviously be a more detailed and complex process than merely conducting a brief interview or consultation at which information is a one way process from the 'professional' to the patient.

Also where there is a lack of adequate social support or the likelihood of non-compliance, these should be considered as equally
important contra-indications to day surgery as is the physically
unfit patient. Patients who have difficulty in grasping the importance of pre-operative fasting or those patients who have undergone
surgery in the past, with no after-effects, will often refuse to
arrange for escorts or carers in the post-operative period because
they are sure that 'they will be fine on their own'. These patients
should be offered in-patient treatment if necessary.

Box 5.1 provides some indicators of the most important areas to
cover during the assessment. Each of these must be discussed with
every patient to reduce the risk of poor outcome and patient
dissatisfaction with day surgery.

THE NURSE'S ROLE IN PROVIDING INFORMATION

As the previous section suggests, nurses can play an important
part in helping patients to understand the implications of their
treatment.

Redman (1988) has shown how the patient education process can
be marked by steps in the nursing process (see Fig. 5.1). She says
that it is possible to educate patients at the same time as carrying
out the other components of the nursing process.

Skilled communication and effective patient education are now an
integral part of effective modern nursing practice, and not confined
solely to the day surgery situation. This was not always recognised
in the past and many nurses did not consider that they were
responsible for providing procedure specific information to their
patients. They felt that this kind of information lay firmly within
the domain of the medical profession.

It is now recognised that nurses contribute significantly towards
patient information and education. Much of the pre-assessment
for day surgery is considered the nurse's responsibility. Most
surgeons and anaesthetists readily acknowledge that adequate
teaching time and effective education for day surgery patients

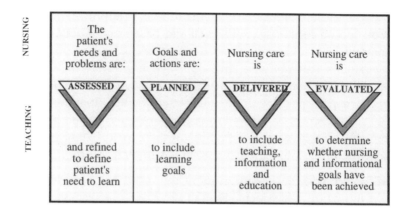

Fig. 5.1   Matching patient teaching needs to the processes of nursing.

can be organised and delivered by experienced out-patient and day surgery nurses.

The nursing assessment interview should not be used solely for selection purposes. It must incorporate verbal information exchange and the opportunity to reinforce written information pitched at a level which is clear and free from medical jargon. Preparing patients and bridging the inevitable knowledge gaps in a timely and structured way will improve the chances of a successful outcome. Good preparation facilitates a trouble-free recovery with less likelihood of unpleasant or unexpected surprises. Nurses can and do play an invaluable part in addressing the gaps which patients are bound to display in their understanding of the day surgery procedure.

CONFORMITY AND CONSISTENCY OF INFORMATION

Before the importance of information to day surgery patients was fully appreciated, nurses were already trying to fill gaps in patient's knowledge informally. They perceived that these important gaps lay in their patient's lack of understanding about this relatively new form of care.

Box 5.2 **Some questions patients may ask about day surgery**

- Who will perform the operation, a consultant or junior doctor?

- Will I have a general anaesthetic or a local anaesthetic?

- How much notice of admission am I going to be given?

- Where will the operation happen?

- What preparation is needed before the day of the operation (and is this different for a day case compared to an in-patient)?

- How long will I be in for (what does a day mean)?

- What do I have to bring with me/wear/eat/not do?

- Do I have to be brought in by somebody else?

- Who do I contact if there's a problem before the admission date? (e.g. if the pain gets worse or if I can't keep the booking)

- What happens if I am not well enough to go home on the day?

- Are there any special arrangements for children? (e.g. eating or drinking before admission, will they be with other children, or adults, can I stay with my child during the day)

Taken from section 1 of **Day Surgery**, Report by the Day Surgery Task Force (Department of Health 1993a).

It gradually became clear that it was possible to anticipate the nature of basic information which would be required and to provide consistent, relevant written and verbal information for all patients. This was relatively straightforward as many patients asked similar questions and often required reassurance in the same areas.

This was acknowledged by the Day Surgery Task Force (Department of Health 1993a) and some of the more frequent questions asked have been reproduced here to illustrate this (see box 5.2).

To ensure that the multi-disciplinary team gives consistent information to patients, time must be set aside for detailed discussion and consultation at the early planning stage. Time spent in formally consulting and agreeing the nature and content of patient information is never wasted; GPs should also be consulted at this stage. Agreeing consistent structured and semi-structured verbal information with all the key players in day surgery will minimise the possibility of patients receiving ambiguous messages. All written material provided should be a collaborative effort for the same reason.

Because surgical practice and anaesthetic technique is continually changing and evolving, particularly in day surgery, a programme which regularly updates all informational material is advisable and again must always involve the whole disciplinary team.

PATIENTS' RIGHTS

Part of the current emphasis on better provision of information within the health service can be attributed to the Patient's Charter which provides more explicit definitions of the rights of the 'consumer' or patient (Department of Health 1995). The Charter explains that patients have the right to be fully informed and will receive clear explanations about the proposed treatment, and alternatives, before agreeing to it (p. 7).

It is to be welcomed that patients are expecting to be provided with more information, especially as they now spend briefer periods in contact with health professionals and must begin to take more responsibility for their own health care needs. There is also evidence that people are adopting a more enquiring attitude to health care. This could be directly attributed to publicity through the Patient's Charter, and higher consumer awareness through the media. Health professionals must address this by focusing their attention more upon treating patients as partners with a role to play in their own care.

COMMUNICATION SKILLS FOR EFFECTIVE INFORMATION EXCHANGE

Sharing information, providing health education and organising effective collaborative programmes toward promoting health have been identified in 'A Vision for the Future' as increasingly important components in all nursing practice (Department of Health 1993b).

Although there is a difference between information, education and teaching, these terms can be used interchangeably under the heading of 'interactive processes' (Brearley 1990). It would be reasonable to assume that the desired outcome of self-care will be achieved by patients who have been adequately informed to take on their own care through the process of education.

Opportunities for teaching can occur at any time during nurse/patient contact and it is important that these opportunities are not wasted but utilised even for casual, unstructured teaching. However, if the barriers to effective teaching and learning are to be minimised, there are a number of strategies which will need to be devised and learned in order to provide as much information as practicable in the best possible way, and over the shortest period of time.

Interactive skill, or communication, implies a two-way process where success depends as much on listening and observing as it does on speaking. The skills which are needed for patient teaching and education need to be learned like any other technical skill. The difference in day surgery is that these skills have to be applied within a very short time-frame. Breaking the process down into the following categories may help.

Communication skills

Non-verbal

Observing non-verbal messages, body language and eye movement, will provide valuable clues as to how a patient is feeling. Non-verbal skills are an integral part of good verbal interview technique. Eye contact, on the same physical level as the patient, a friendly handshake and careful thought in the placing of furniture, even the decoration in an interview room, will all assist in good communication by reducing sensory overload and anxiety which is nearly always associated with a hospital visit.

Verbal

It is important to speak clearly, without using medical jargon, to listen attentively and to ask open-ended questions. Open-ended questions usually help to ensure that more useful information is forthcoming than merely a 'yes' or 'no'.

When imparting information it is helpful to pause frequently. This will give the patient the opportunity to interrupt and to ask for clarification. By listening to what a patient says, the nurse can collect important clues about levels of understanding. Subsequent conversation can then be pitched at the level which a patient will more readily understand.

Some suggestions regarding the possible conduct of a preoperative interview are given below.

Begin by determining what the patient already knows:

'You have just been to see the surgeon, what did he tell you about your operation?'

Start with simple explanations. Explain the most important points first and then gradually move to the more complex:

'You will be coming into hospital just for the day but you will be having a general anaesthetic (that is, you will be given an injection to make you sleep while you are operated on). This has some after-effects and means you must take time to recover and you must have someone to take you home and stay with you at home until the effects wear off....'

'The operation you are having may mean that you will have some pain afterward, but we will give you something to help with that....'

Ask the patient to interrupt if the information is not clear:

'Do tell me if you are not clear about your day case operation and please stop me if I am going too quickly or you need anything clarified....'

Reinforce the conversation with some pertinent written information. Use it as a framework for the interview:

'Most of what you need to know is in this information leaflet which I shall give you. It explains first what a general anaesthetic is and how you need to prepare for it and then goes on to explain the procedure for when you arrive. . . .'

'I will also give you an information leaflet which explains your operation and tells you what you should do to recover comfortably at home. . . .'

Finish with a resumé of the important points:

'I have explained what time you should arrive, how to prepare for your anaesthetic and what your surgical procedure is about. Are there any points which are not clear?'

'Please remember how important it is for you to have a responsible escort, that you must not drive yourself home and that you should have someone at home to take care of things while you recover.'

'You can contact us between now and your operation day by telephone if you think of anything else you need to ask.'

Determining information deficits

It is important that the questionnaire which determines safe physical patient selection is completed by the patient at a pre-assessment interview which is not too long before the intended admission date. It may not be possible at this time to determine the level of knowledge of carers. These carers assume a high level of responsibility for their charges recovering at home from surgery and general anaesthesia, considerably greater than for the more conventional surgical admission. Much more is expected of them in terms of support, care and their attendance during the first 24–48 hours at home. It is therefore advisable to provide a leaflet which explains their part in the proceedings.

See Chapter 3, Table 3.1, for question-naire

The opportunity may present itself at this stage for health education, by explaining the effect of smoking at the same time as providing the reason for abstention before a general anaesthesia.

However, day surgery nurses will obviously need to come to terms with some of the limitations which the constraints of lack of time and brief contact with patients impose upon them. Even if there was sufficient time, it may be unrealistic to expect day surgery patients to absorb many of the complex issues surrounding health promotion or education involving fundamental changes in their life-style. It is important to remember that the information which nurses do provide to day patients should be clearly focused on teaching about the present episode of care.

Some simple additional questions here could help to determine gaps in understanding and can be used to augment a patient's knowledge. Some examples of these are illustrated below:

Do you know what operation you will be having as a day case?

IF THE ANSWER IS YES:
ensure knowledge is accurate and provide procedure-specific information to read at home.

IF NO:
explain in detail and provide procedure-specific information to read at home.

Will this be your first operation?

IF THE ANSWER IS YES:
explain exactly what happens and how to prepare.

IF NO:
find out in what setting this took place and explain what is different about a day surgery operation and how to prepare.

Have you ever had any reactions to anaesthetics?

IF THE ANSWER IS YES:
explain the difference between day case and in-patient anaesthesia, the importance of fasting and how to recuperate at home safely and comfortably.

IF NO:
explain what is different about day surgery anaesthesia and the importance of fasting and taking time to recover before driving, returning to work etc.

Will you have to go home alone?

IF THE ANSWER IS YES:
explain that it will not then be possible to have day case surgery unless a suitable adult escort can be found. Explain the importance of private car for comfort and that the back of a motor bike will not do!

IF NO:
explain why it is important to have someone to drive home by car and to stay for the first 24–48 hours because of the effects of anaesthesia (these can be explained in more detail here).

Do you know how long it is advisable to recuperate before resuming normal activity?

IF THE ANSWER IS YES:
ensure knowledge is accurate and discuss normal symptoms after an operation.

IF NO:
explain in detail and reinforce the importance of taking time to recover even though surgery may appear to have been minor.

Do you have a telephone?

IF THE ANSWER IS YES:
give details about who to contact if symptoms appear to be abnormal and explain what these might be.

IF NO:
explain that it would be advisable to reschedule surgery for an overnight stay to avoid complications occurring with no means of obtaining advice or support.

As the above questions illustrate, a few well-chosen and strategic enquiries can lead to important exchanges of information and the development of a deeper discussion which should help to clarify the patient's knowledge and will reinforce their ability to cope.

Printed information

Individuals may not always read at the level of their completed formal education (Redman 1988). Written material should be pitched at a level which will be easily understood by the lay person. It should avoid obscure medical jargon and terms which could be ambiguous.

Following a few simple principles in compiling written information leaflets can ensure that they are 'user friendly' and at a level which most people can understand. Consider the need to translate material into other languages and explore the possibility of cassette or video information for people with special needs. Having written the information, use the following general criteria to check it:

- Sentences should be no more than 15 to 20 words long.

- Words used should be no more than three syllables long.

- Avoid jargon, slang and vague or inaccurate expressions (such as 'rupture' instead of 'hernia' or 'put to sleep' instead of 'general anaesthetic').

- Medical terms should be explained immediately in the text.

- Personalise the leaflet by referring to the patient as 'you'.

- Avoid too many words ending in -ion (i.e. 'this leaflet explains your hernia repair' is preferable to 'this is an explanation about hernia repair).

- Always include a contact telephone number for enquiries.

- Use print which can easily be read (this should be mandatory for ophthalmic day cases).

- Consider printing or desk top publishing rather than using a poor quality photocopier.

Two examples of procedure-specific information leaflets (on wisdom teeth removal and diagnostic laparoscopy) are provided in Tables 5.1 and 5.2. They could be reproduced or altered to suit the local needs of any day surgery unit.

More general information for all patients in day surgery should accompany the procedure-specific leaflet and must be carefully designed and consistent in content. This information will need to contain detailed information about the following:

■ how to prepare for general anaesthesia, if appropriate;

■ what time to arrive;

■ what time surgery will take place;

■ what time to tell an escort to arrive and how long someone should stay with them at home after their surgery;

■ what arrangements will be made for pain relief and dressings, if necessary;

■ how to recognise an emergency, what to do and who to contact;

■ why it is important not to drive, operate machinery or make important decisions while under the influence of a general anaesthetic or sedation (for 24 to 48 hours);

■ how long it would be advisable to recuperate before resuming normal activity;

■ what arrangements will be made for follow-up care.

Written information about the more general arrangements for admission and specific information about the actual procedure (with space to add or reinforce any special instructions), should be provided well in advance. It is preferable to be able to discuss this with the patient. If it needs to be sent by post, an accompanying letter should state that any further questions will be welcomed. Figure 5.2 provides a basic outline of the kind of format which written information might take. It is important to vary the text and style and icons can help to draw the eye towards the important messages which need to be read and understood.

Table 5.1   **Sample patient information I**

Post-operative information after removal of your WISDOM TEETH
You may experience some discomfort, swelling and bruising, but this should resolve after a few days. If you have had a local anaesthetic your mouth may be numb for a time. After surgery you should avoid hot drinks and eating hot foods for the first day.

Oral hygiene
After all meals and last thing at night you should use hot salt mouthwashes (a half a teaspoon of salt or a measure of mouthwash in a tumblerful of hot water). This will help to keep your mouth clean and prevent infection. Start this the day after your operation. You should also brush your teeth as normal, twice daily and after meals starting the day after your operation.

Antibiotics
You may be given some antibiotic tablets to prevent infection which should be taken as directed on the bottle. Alcohol should be avoided if you are given Metronidazole. Those on the contraceptive pill should also use other contraceptive protection for the whole month, as some antibiotics may prevent the pill from working effectively.

Pain control
A mild analgesic (pain killer) such as paracetamol or codeine is helpful. You may be given a stronger analgesic for the first few days, such as Ibuprofen 400 mg which should be taken every six hours.

Smoking and exercise
You are advised not to take any strenuous exercise for 24 hours and to stop smoking for 48 hours.

Bleeding
If bleeding occurs once you have left the hospital, roll up a clean cotton handkerchief and use this to bite on the operation site for 20 minutes and the bleeding should stop. Do not disturb the handkerchief during this time.

Sutures
The surgery may require sutures (stitches) in the mouth, these are usually reabsorbable and dissolve or are dislodged with cleaning the teeth after about a week. They should not need to be removed.

General anaesthesia
After a general anaesthetic you may feel tired and experience muscular aches and pains. This discomfort resolves after 48 hours and is helped by taking paracetamol or similar analgesia (painkiller).

If you require further advice
If at any time you have a problem, please contact:
The duty Oral Surgeon at the hospital on
(Tel. No.   )

You may also ring the day surgery unit on
(Tel. No.   ) for advice
between 8 a.m. and 6 p.m.

Table 5.2 **Sample patient information II**

DIAGNOSTIC LAPAROSCOPY

What is a laparoscopy?

A laparoscopy is the examination of your lower internal organs by means of a small telescope (about the diameter of a pencil). Through the telescope the surgeon can see your uterus, ovaries and fallopian tubes as well as all the other structures within your pelvis. The laparoscope is introduced through a very small incision, usually just below your tummy button. Occasionally another incision, about the same size, will be made to obtain a better view of those organs lower down in your pelvis.

How will I feel afterwards?

You may wake from your anaesthetic with a little abdominal discomfort. You will normally have been given an injection of a fairly strong painkiller before you awake. If you find it difficult to rest it is sensible to ask for further pain relief and this can usually be given orally once you are awake.

Just occasionally you may experience some discomfort in your neck and shoulders. This is caused by some air which was introduced into your abdomen during the operation, which helps to obtain a better view. Most of this air is dispersed before the end of the operation but sometimes a little may lodge beneath your diaphragm causing some upward pressure. This will be absorbed, usually in the 24 hours after your operation, and you will be given some tablets to take home which should relieve the discomfort.

How long will it take to get back to normal?

After your operation you will want to rest quietly in your bed (or trolley) until late afternoon. When you go home you will be advised to go to bed and rest for at least 24 hours. (Some people do require a little longer). Your surgeon will advise you before you leave hospital as to when you should resume your usual routine.

Are there any complications with this operation?

Very occasionally your surgeon may find it necessary to extend your operation into a slightly more major procedure if he has any difficulty in seeing your pelvic organs through the telescope. This will mean a slightly longer stay in hospital to recover.

There should be very little bleeding from your little wound(s) and it is rare for you to get any infection in them. You may experience a little bleeding from the vagina but this should not be as heavy as an ordinary period.

Is there anything else I should know?

You will see your surgeon after your operation and he/she will inform you of the arrangements to follow you up in the out-patient clinic. These arrangements will be made in the day surgery unit and your appointment will reach you by mail soon after you get home. (Please contact us if you do not receive it within a week to ten days after your visit.)

You should not return to work until you feel 'back to normal'. The anaesthetic will take 24 hours to leave your system, so do not undertake any task which requires fine coordination or might be dangerous.

Your stitches (if any) will dissolve by themselves and you may bath normally and leave your wound(s) without a dressing unless you find them 'catching' on your underwear. It is advisable not to spend too long in a bath for the first week, just in case your stitches dissolve before the healing process is completed.

Please contact us if you require any further help on (Tel. No. ....) between 7.30 a.m. and 6 p.m. (Mon–Fri). You may also wish to contact your GP if you are worried about anything. It is possible to contact the Gynaecology Registrar through the main hospital switchboard (Tel. No. ....).

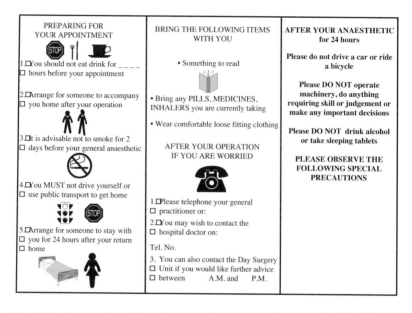

Fig. 5.2 A sample design for a patient pre-admission leaflet. The package must also include procedure-specific information, a map and a programme of what will happen on the day.

Reinforcing and evaluating information

The adequacy and successful assimilation of information and teaching material can be determined by assessing the compliance and understanding of patients. Patients will frequently require some reinforcement of the information they are given because of the strange surroundings or anxiety experienced when first confronted with the possibility of an operation.

To evaluate the effectiveness of information a process of continuous audit should address whether patients are receiving and assimilating adequate information. This can be monitored from the occasions when patients arrive unprepared, need further explanation or experience difficulty at home (elicited from a follow-up telephone call, see Chapter 4).

See Chapter 4

If patients arrive unprepared and ignorant about what is to happen to them, then obviously the teaching method is not working. This evaluation of patient compliance should be used to tailor information more specifically to the needs of patients for the future.

THE BALANCE BETWEEN WRITTEN AND VERBAL INFORMATION

Because of the time constraint, it could be tempting to rely too heavily on standard written information. There are significant reasons why this means of educating or teaching patients alone is flawed. Written information can never properly address the unique and individual needs of each patient as effectively as a structured verbal interview. Also there is no guarantee that written information will be read or assimilated adequately without the help of verbal reinforcement.

The most effective way to exchange information is to use the assessment interview as a means of providing essential information, using the written material to prompt any additional clarification or questions from the patient. This will usually draw out the most important information gaps which need to be addressed.

CONCLUSION

Every nurse in day surgery needs to assess the ability of patients to cope with their own care but it is, perhaps, unrealistic to expect them to do much more than provide fairly basic information. Nor will they be able to assess and address every individual knowledge deficit in each patient in the time available. Time, a valuable commodity in day surgery, will never be wasted if it can be used to determine what the patient knows and then to fill the most important gaps in their knowledge.

There is obviously much more extensive and detailed guidance elsewhere in the literature about how to go about providing comprehensive patient information and education. This chapter has focused upon the more practical aspects of delivering important information to day surgery patients in the short time available. It is obviously not intended to be a substitute to further study and reading on the subject.

ACTION GUIDELINES

- to recognise, identify and address knowledge deficits at an early stage and to understand the importance of clear, consistent information for the self-caring patient.

- to use information as a means to minimise the risk of poor outcome and to increase compliance

- to understand the nurses role, as part of the day surgery team, in providing agreed consistent general and procedure-specific information to day patients

- to analyse some communication strategies and to evaluate the effectiveness of the information provided to day surgery patients

Further reading

KEMPE, A.R. (1987) Patient education for the ambulatory surgery patient. *AORN Journal* **45**, no. 2 pp. 500–506. Lists some useful teaching strategies and plans for day case teaching, and discusses the use of audio and video material.

PALM, M.L. (1971) Recognising opportunities for informal patient teaching. *Nursing Clinics of North America* **94**, pp. 669–678. Discusses and identifies when is the best time for patient teaching. Emphasises the importance of using every available opportunity for teaching

REDMAN, B.K. (1988) **The Process of Patient Education**. C.V. Mosby, St Louis. Provides definitions, models and current practices in patient teaching. Provides in-depth text on patient motivation to learn and the importance of patient education.

RICE, V. & JOHNSON, J. (1984) Pre-admission self-instruction booklets, post-admission exercise performance and teaching time. *Nursing Research*, **33**, pp. 147–151. A study into the effects of pre-operative teaching upon the post-operative recovery of patients.

References

BREARLEY, S. (1990) **Patient Participation: The Literature**. Scutari Press, Harrow.

DEPARTMENT OF HEALTH (1993a) **Day Surgery**, Report by the Day Surgery Task Force. NHS – Management Executive, HMSO, London.

DEPARTMENT OF HEALTH (1993b) **A Vision for the Future, The Nursing, Midwifery and Health Visiting Contribution to Health and Health Care.** HMSO, London.

DEPARTMENT OF HEALTH (1995) **NHS – The Patient's Charter and You.** HMSO, London.

GARRAWAY, W.M., CUTHBERTSON, C., FENWICK, N., RUCKLEY, C.V. & PRESCOTT, R.J. (1978) Consumer acceptability of day-care after operations for hernia or varicose veins. *Journal of Epidemiology and Community Health.* **32**, pp. 219–221.

REDMAN, B.K. (1988) **The Process of Patient Education**. C.V. Mosby, St Louis.

Reports of the Health Service Commissioner for England, for Scotland and for Wales: Annual Report for 1994–1995. HMSO, London.

6

The Education of Nurses for Day Surgery

Introduction – Education for day surgery nursing practice – Steps in the day surgery process – Expanding nursing skills – Defining competence – Clinical supervision or preceptorship – Competencies – A competency-based training programme – Conclusion

THIS CHAPTER: Describes the skills required for nursing in an integrated day surgery unit. Nurses who work with day cases in day and in-patient wards, theatres and recovery areas are skilled in these specific areas. It is suggested here that integrated units need a versatile and competent nursing service to manage and co-ordinate the care of patients throughout the whole day surgery process. To achieve this, nurses will need to acquire a comprehensive set of skills or competencies. These competencies are made explicit in this chapter and can be acquired as a planned programme under the tutelage of a preceptor or clinical supervisor to underpin appropriate formal training.

INTRODUCTION

Previous chapters have emphasised the importance of addressing the specific needs of day surgery patients, regardless of where they are nursed. In conventional in-patient settings, the surgical ward nurse cares for patients both before and after surgery while theatre, anaesthetic and recovery nurses take responsibility for anaesthesia and surgical intervention. Subsequently, community and practice nurses will often deliver the required follow-up care.

Day surgery unit nurses have the rewarding role of nursing each patient through the whole day surgery experience. They can also take some responsibility for supporting patients after their discharge by providing verbal and written information and advice once the patient has returned home.

EDUCATION FOR DAY SURGERY NURSING PRACTICE

In view of the increasing number of day surgery facilities being commissioned, it would be impossible to expect all nursing staff to have formally assimilated all the knowledge and skills needed before being appointed to a post in day surgery. Also, formal day surgery nursing courses are expensive and still comparatively rare (A list of centres currently providing these is provided in Appendix 1).

Validation by the English National Board for specific day surgery courses has helped to provide the service with programmes which cover the needs of patients throughout day surgery. These courses emphasise the importance of a theoretical base for holistic care which is far removed from traditional 'task allocation', and the 'theatre course'. It is stressed that, although obviously important, the theatre component represents only a very minor part of day surgical nursing care.

This chapter concentrates on analysing some specific day surgery nursing skills, many but not all of which can be acquired during practice. Each of the competencies described later should be seen solely as a framework around which to develop one of the most rewarding objectives of day surgery, that of 'seamless' nursing care.

A more consistent and efficient service can be provided when one nurse can take responsibility for all or most of a patient's nursing care before, during and after the day surgical process. This can be achieved, in an integrated day surgery unit, by helping nurses to a develop the skills needed in each distinct component of day surgical intervention.

STEPS IN THE DAY SURGERY PROCESS

As Fig 6.1 below shows, a day surgery experience consists of a series of distinct episodes with clearly defined beginning and end points. By regarding each of these steps as discrete components of the whole, each one can be satisfactorily completed. However, they should only be seen as clearly separate episodes by members of the health care team. To the patient the experience should appear to be one continuous episode of care. To achieve this the care ought to be co-ordinated and facilitated by the same nurse throughout the patient's journey through day surgery.

EXPANDING NURSING SKILLS

Surgical nursing has traditionally divided the care of patients into the following separately staffed distinct areas:

- pre-operative preparation,

- operating theatre technique,

- post-operative recovery,

- discharge into community care.

Primary nursing and the named nurse concept is an aspiration for many nurses who work in these settings and there are still some components of care which many 'primary nurses' must still leave to other colleagues.

However, in an integrated unit the day surgery nurse informs, cares for and discharges a group of patients, supporting them through the whole experience. They advise patients and their carers throughout and in the immediate recovery phase to prepare them for discharge. They complete this care with an evaluation process, usually by means of a phone call after a day or two at home.

To achieve this 'seamless' service, the emphasis should be on expanding the competency-based skills of the day surgery nursing workforce. Day surgery managers can facilitate the process by:

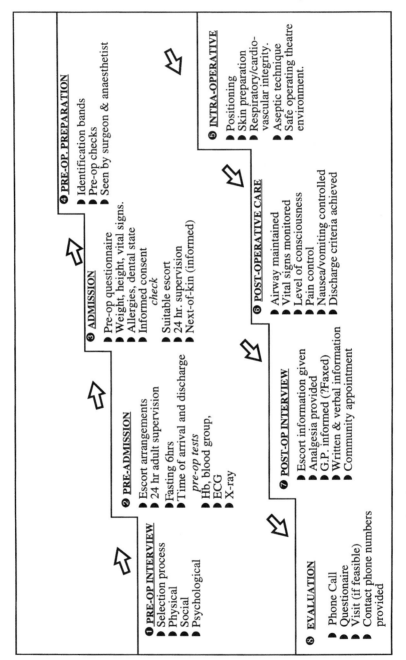

❶ PRE-OP INTERVIEW
- Selection process
- Physical
- Social
- Psychological

❷ PRE-ADMISSION
- Escort arrangements
- 24 hr adult supervision
- Fasting 6hrs
- Time of arrival and discharge
- *pre-op tests*
- Hb, blood group,
- ECG
- X-ray

❸ ADMISSION
- Pre-op questionnaire
- Weight, height, vital signs.
- Allergies, dental state
- Informed consent *check*
- Suitable escort
- 24 hr. supervision
- Next-of-kin (informed)

❹ PRE-OP. PREPARATION
- Identification bands
- Pre-op checks
- Seen by surgeon & anaesthetist

❺ INTRA-OPERATIVE
- Positioning
- Skin preparation
- Respiratory/cardio-vascular integrity.
- Aseptic technique
- Safe operating theatre environment.

❻ POST-OPERATIVE CARE
- Airway maintained
- Vital signs monitored
- Level of consciousness
- Pain control
- Nausea/vomiting controlled
- Discharge criteria achieved

❼ POST-OP INTERVIEW
- Escort information given
- Analgesia provided
- G.P. informed (?Faxed)
- Written & verbal information
- Community appointment

❽ EVALUATION
- Phone Call
- Questionaire
- Visit (if feasible)
- Contact phone numbers provided

Fig. 6.1   The steps in the day surgery process.

- allocating new staff to experienced mentors in each area of day surgery;

- developing a comprehensive programme of supervised practice;

- systematic assessment and documentation of competence.

A well trained, versatile and efficient team, capable of working in the pre-assessment clinic, operating theatre and recovery areas will ensure the smooth running of the unit. This flexibility also helps to avoid the unwelcome, but often familiar, crisis management which is almost inevitable to cover sickness and absence in areas of specialised nursing practice.

DEFINING COMPETENCE

Competence encompasses far more than merely the ability to carry out physical care or efficient technical skills. It embraces knowledge, skill, values, beliefs and attitudes, all of which underpin effective nursing practice.

An explicit philosophy for nursing can provide the foundation upon which to build competence. Commonly held beliefs, or philosophy, are formulated to help nurses articulate what they know intuitively. A philosophy can be written by:

See Chapter 4 for a philosophy of nursing in day surgery

- explaining the particular characteristics of a group of patients;

- describing the effects which treatment will have upon them;

- identifying why nursing care is required to ameliorate the effects and at particular times of need;

- describing the ideal environment and resources required for effective nursing to take place.

CLINICAL SUPERVISION OR PRECEPTORSHIP

A system of preceptorship, clinical supervision or mentorship from an expert, experienced nurse can guide inexperienced nurses towards achieving accountability and personal competency in their chosen field of nursing. Benner (1984) found that clinical expertise is particularly influenced by experience, especially in similar patient populations. A formal structure of preceptorship will facilitate teaching for the 'beginning' nurse and for the experienced nurse who transfers to a new area.

Any formal educational programme for day surgery nursing should begin with discrete periods of clinical supervision from an experienced nurse. Clinical supervision is high on nursing's agenda as a means of promoting good practice. It has been described by Butterworth and Faugier (1992) as 'an exchange between practising professionals to enable the development of professional skills'. Once supervisors (and their supervisees) are trained they can begin to work collaboratively, outside management hierarchies, to promote effective practice, exercise accountability and reflect on clinical expertise. As the system becomes established it should encourage reflection, review the effectiveness of nursing practice to a level which a managerial system of performance review has not yet generally succeeded in reaching.

Realistically, it is probably true to say that clinical supervision will be easier to administer in established day surgery units where nurses are infrequently appointed. It will be more difficult in a new day surgery unit where appointments are made *en masse*. Supervision from an experienced practitioner from outside the unit may need to be arranged and this should be considered early in the planning stage.

COMPETENCIES

The competencies outlined in this chapter are intended as a guide for training nurses to work confidently within all the areas which make up their day surgery unit.

When nurses join the team they will need to identify their existing skills and knowledge and negotiate help for those upon which they need to build. An individually tailored programme of preceptorship or supervision, using these competencies, will therefore meet some of their training needs. Box 6.1 below lists the basic skills which should be acquired by the newly appointed nurse.

Box 6.1 Specific skills for day surgery

- Pre-operative preparation

- Selection and assessment

- Counselling skills

- Teaching and educating patients and their carers

- Admission assessment

- Operating theatre technique and management

- Recovery-room care

- Discharge arrangement and evaluation

Before a system of clinical supervision is implemented all new staff must be supported by a suitable period of 'in service' education and orientation, under the supervision of an experienced nurse. A team of nurses who are proficient in all areas in the unit should become mentors for as long as necessary to support new staff. All newly recruited staff should be given time to work through the whole system under this expert guidance until they are judged proficient.

If staff are recruited from areas of surgical nursing, and have gained some expertise, they will immediately feel comfortable performing familiar tasks. However, they should be supported and encouraged to achieve competency in the other areas, as much as possible at their own pace, while continuing as useful members of staff in the areas where they feel most 'at home'.

A COMPETENCY-BASED TRAINING PROGRAMME

The following set of competencies is designed to cover the whole day surgical process. They are, however, merely a framework to guide the day surgery manager who wishes to provide a structured educational programme for new day surgery nurses.

As previously explained, each of these competencies can be worked through with an experienced mentor and should be 'signed off' during a suitable period of induction.

Every nurse who joins the team will almost certainly arrive with some educational needs. Some will already possess expertise in some areas of conventional surgical nursing but many will identify gaps in their knowledge about the specific needs of day surgery patients. It was for this reason that this particular set of competencies was developed.

Competency one

Box 6.2 Competency one: Nurses will be able to screen and assist in the suitable selection of patients for day surgical procedures by:

- identifying suitable surgical procedures for day surgery and providing specific advice to patients on these

- liaising with relevant clinicians, as appropriate, to determine selection guidelines

- having an 'in depth' understanding of selection guidelines and an understanding of the rationale for working within them

- being aware of different referral methods to day surgery

- co-ordinating pre-operative screening investigations which may be relevant to the procedure

- communicating effectively with patients to explain selection criteria and providing all necessary information and guidance prior to admission

---

Important elements within Competency one

■ Screening patients to determine their suitability for a day surgery procedure is probably the most critical element of all the factors which will contribute to a successful outcome to day surgery.

■ It is important that day surgery nurses become proficient in recognising potential social, psychological, surgical or anaesthetic complications which may have been missed in a busy out-patient department. Anticipation of some of the less obvious contra-indications to day surgery avoids the possibility of patients arriving on the day of surgery, only to face unexpected delays or a last-minute cancellation.

■ Many patients are able to attend a day surgery facility for selection, screening and information, with obvious benefits. However, geographical and operational factors sometimes make this impossible. A number of different people, therefore, might be involved in the referral process. They need to be aware of the strict selection criteria so as to communicate these properly to patients who cannot attend for pre-assessment. If a pre-assessment system is not in operation, therefore, it is crucial that the day surgery nurse maintain regular contact with the relevant referring colleagues within, for example:

■ Out-patient departments,
■ Outreach clinics,
■ Consultants' offices,
■ Wards,
■ General practitioner surgeries,
■ Primary health care facilities.

■ As nurses gain experience, they should be able take the responsibility for conducting the patient assessment and for making informed decisions about the selection of patients. Obviously they must work within clearly agreed and explicit guidelines and any uncertainty or alteration to these needs will need to be communicated and agreed. Nursing screening and selection will only be effective if the selection criteria remain consistent or are altered with the agreement of all concerned.

- The nurse also needs to be able to define the difference between minor and intermediate procedures and will be aware of the different anaesthetic techniques which are most appropriate for specific day surgery procedures.

Competency two

Box 6.3 **Competency two: Nurses will assess and plan care for each individual patient by:**

- establishing a rapport with the patient to elicit appropriate information and developing good communication skills

- recognising the psychosocial effects of day surgical treatment upon individual patients and their carers

- acting in partnership with patients to increase awareness and understanding about the effects of anaesthetic and surgical intervention

- evaluating, documenting and communicating physiological health status

Important elements within Competency two

- Nurses should be able to build upon their ability to assess, plan and implement patient care, learnt in other settings. More importantly, perhaps, they will need to 'fine tune' their communication skills in view of the limited time available to make effective patient contact.

- The psychological barriers to a successful outcome must be assessed and strategies planned to alleviate these. The absolute necessity for good social support is a crucial element in all patient assessment for day surgery, which is not always fully appreciated or anticipated, particularly in in-patient settings. Nurses also need to assess patient suitability in the light of demographic factors, the particular needs of different patient populations and for specific client groups.

■ Patients need to be made aware of the significant factors which determine their selection, or otherwise, for day surgery. Before they consent to this method of treatment, they must be given clear, unambiguous information. It has already been stressed that this can only be achieved if nurses and clinicians can communicate consistent, previously agreed, information to patients and their carers. See Chapter 5

■ Although a surgeon and anaesthetist take primary responsibility for determining physiological health status, the nurse should describe the practical aspects of the effects of anaesthesia and surgery in greater depth to both the patient and his or her carer.

■ Planning and documenting care should include details about the current health status of the patient and clear information about their specific needs. The nurse should be able to formulate, with the patient, an appropriate plan of care. Very often the patient will assist with this and, to streamline the process and save time, the health status questionnaire can become the basic framework for a care plan. See Chapter 3, Table 3.1

■ Practical nursing skills will also be required for the measurement and recording of vital signs accurately, and to recognise and report any deviations from the norm. All relevant changes in health status since the initial pre-assessment must be noted on admission, and medication, allergies and adverse reactions established.

Competency three

> ### Box 6.4 Competency three: Nurses will be able to care for patients undergoing all forms of anaesthesia relevant to day surgery by:
>
> ■ possessing an in-depth knowledge of the different forms and effects of anaesthesia
>
> ■ co-ordinating the pre-operative screening and relevant investigations required for anaesthesia
>
> ■ delivering effective nursing care to patient undergoing all forms of anaesthesia

Important elements within Competency three

■ Day surgery general anaesthesia is usually tailored to the specific conditions required for a rapid recovery and for minimal residual post-operative after-effects. There are effective combinations of intravenous, inhalation, regional and local anaesthetic blockade which can provide a comfortable and pain-free recovery period. These are constantly being refined and are the subject of much recent research. Nurses may need to refer to the literature to become well-informed and up-to-date in the changing aspects and nature of anaesthetic technique.

See Further reading at the end of this chapter

■ The nurse will often take some of the responsibility for organising relevant blood tests, X-rays and appropriate investigations, if necessary. Results must be available within an acceptable time before anaesthesia to avoid a last-minute delay or cancellation of an operation. If they are to take on this responsibility and to interpret the results properly, nurses will need to possess a good working knowledge of physiological norms.

■ If nurses are to support and guide patients throughout the perioperative period, they will need to understand and recognise the specific stages of anaesthesia. It is important, too, for accurate explanations to be conveyed to patient and carer, since they also must recognise what are the normal and abnormal post-operative symptoms after discharge home.

Competency four (Box 6.5)

Important elements within Competency four

■ Not all nurses have the desire or the aptitude to work in the operating room. It is a matter of some debate as to whether nurses need to become proficient in these purely technical areas. However, they do need to enforce the safeguards and protocols which are designed to ensure the safety of patients in the operating room, and also take responsibility for patient care while patients are unable to take care of themselves.

Box 6.5 **Competency four: Nurses will be able to create a safe environment throughout invasive procedures by:**

- preparing the operating room, instrumentation, apparatus and equipment with regard for safety and comfort of the patient

- possessing a good working knowledge of, checking and preparing regularly maintained anaesthetic and monitoring equipment

- positioning patients to ensure safety and comfort

- maintaining strict aseptic technique and ensuring clean conditions and the use of sterilised equipment

- acting as circulating nurse during procedures

- acting as 'scrub nurse' within the operating team

- The maintenance and upkeep of the day surgery unit should be of the same high standard as an in-patient facility. The nurse must become proficient in lifting and handling techniques and safe positioning of the patient, however short the procedure. Because of the speed of throughput in day surgery, there is a constant temptation to 'cut corners' and this must be avoided at all costs.

- The principles of asepsis should be familiar to all nurses but performing this at speed is not always easy. Where there are large numbers of patients treated at speed, there can be major problems finding the time to teach new members of staff to become manually dextrous, to act as circulating nurse and in scrubbing techniques. It is worth considering a period of secondment to an in-patient operating theatre, for two reasons. The pace is slower there and major surgery will give the nurse some confidence in dealing with what are inevitable but unexpected complications in the day surgery unit.

Competency five

Box 6.6   Competency five: Nurses are able to undertake full nursing care of the patient during the immediate recovery phase by:

■ undertaking total nursing care of patients until recovery from unconsciousness is complete

■ monitoring and maintaining homeostasis, vital signs and patient airway

■ effectively managing respiratory and cardiac emergency

■ regularly updating knowledge and performance for cardio-pulmonary resuscitation

Important elements within Competency five

■ It is important to emphasise to inexperienced nurses in day surgery that there is no such thing as a 'minor' general anaesthetic. The recovery of patients in day surgery can be as fraught with danger as any in-patient procedure and the ability to act quickly and confidently must be appreciated.

■ All the necessary recovery equipment should be available and the nurse needs to become familiar with using it. While patients may not be intubated, they can still experience respiratory difficulty and any number of complications associated with drug interaction and anaesthetic or surgical intervention.

Competency six (Box 6.7)

Important elements within Competency six

■ It requires experience for a nurse to make decisions about patient discharge when some post-operative symptoms persist. Pain, nausea, vomiting and dizziness should obviously be adequately controlled but patients may remain drowsy for some hours and discharge home might ensure that they will settle better and rest to overcome this.

Box 6.7 **Competency six: Nurses will be able to educate patients to return home safely to recover in their own environment by:**

- assessing that vital signs conform to original baseline observations

- ensuring that nausea or vomiting are treated

- ensuring that pain is adequately controlled and that provision is made for appropriate analgesia to take home

- ensuring that adequate social support is available

- providing written discharge instructions with verbal reinforcement of a general and specific nature

- co-ordinating community liaison, follow-up care and contact telephone numbers

- Verbal and written communication of discharge advice to a responsible escort is vital to ensure suitable after-care arrangements. Nurses should have insight into the home circumstances where patients will be recovering. They should be able to advise on the best way to ensure a comfortable recovery and to arrange for back-up support and community assistance, where necessary. They should become able to recognise where a patient might require some extra support and reassurance, which may not be considered necessary from a strictly medical viewpoint.

- Nurses will need to learn to determine when it would be advisable to seek an in-patient overnight bed for a patient who does not recover sufficiently in time to return home. There should be no sense of failure if a patient is deemed unfit to return home and, often, a few hours longer to recover is all that is needed. It is important to ensure that nurses know how to provide emotional support and satisfactory explanations to patient and carer when things have not gone according to plan. Obviously a fully documented record of operative procedure, type of anaesthesia and post-operative management will also need to be communicated to ward staff.

Competency seven

Box 6.8   Competency seven: Nurses will be able to evaluate satisfactory outcome by:

- determining that patients meet discharge criteria before discharge

- ensuring that pain control is effective and fully understood

- monitoring patient and carer satisfaction through patient satisfaction surveys and research into all aspects of patient activity in day surgery

- arranging good follow-up arrangements, emergency contact numbers and telephoning patients to determine recovery process after discharge

---

Important elements within Competency seven

See also
Chapter 2,
Box 2.7

- Teaching discharge criteria to nurses serves two main purposes. They will provide a valuable 'checklist' to remind nurses about what physical capabilities they should be assessing to determine if patients can safely return home. They can also be utilised as an evaluation tool and will provide written documentary proof of a patient's fitness for discharge.

- Pain control must be effective and, obviously, not only while patients are in hospital. It is important to teach nurses how to inform patients about methods to achieve pain control at home and to ensure that written information accompanies them home. Additional advice should be given about what to do if they cannot control their pain themselves.

- Nurses must be able to appreciate the need to adapt information to take account of the individual needs and abilities of their patients. Follow-up arrangements should be adapted and individualised to suit each patient. Evaluation of the care provided and post-operative progress can be determined, either by questionnaire, a phone call or both.

See also Chapter 4, Box 4.2

CONCLUSION

Educating nurses using the framework provided by these peri-operative competencies will help all concerned in the care of day patients to appreciate the innovative and challenging nature of this form of care. Also, they will, perhaps, better equip themselves to meet the specific needs of the short-stay patient. As has been emphasised in previous chapters, these patients have different and, perhaps, greater educational and informational needs because of the shorter periods of contact they have with health professionals.

The competencies described in this chapter are by no means exhaustive and are intended only to provide a template for an experienced nurse to use for the induction and education of newly appointed nurses. Wherever possible, and where resources permit, they should be used in conjunction with other educational strategies and underpinned with more formal teaching programmes.

ACTION GUIDELINES

- Develop both formal and practice-based teaching in day surgery

- Take the lead in implementing a system of preceptorship and clinical supervision for nursing staff

- Appreciate the professional advantages of a structured approach to induction of new staff to day surgery

- Study the competencies set out in this chapter and consider using them as a framework for teaching day surgery practice

Further reading

NURSING STANDARD (1994) **8**, No. 52. Clinical practice development: Preparing to take on clinical supervision. Discusses the importance of clinical supervision, and outlines how nurses can introduce the concept into practice.

UKCC (1996) Position statement on clinical supervision for nursing and health visiting. UKCC, London. Sets out the definition and suggestions for models of clinical supervision in nursing practice.

NHS Management Executive (1993) **Day Surgery**, Report by the Day Surgery Task Force. A shortened version of competencies can be found in the Day Surgery Task Force Report, contributed by the author of this handbook.

CAMPBELL, W.I. (1990) Analgesic side effects and minor surgery. *British Journal of Anaesthesia* **64**, pp. 617–620. The use of non-steroidals and analgesia is advantageous in reducing the need for stronger opioids for day surgery.

SMITH, I., VAN HEMELRIJCK, J., WHITE, P.F. & SHIVELY, R. (1991) Effects of local anaesthesia on recovery after out-patient arthoscopy. *Anaesthesia Analgesia* **73**, pp. 536–539. Effects of local anaesthesia on recovery after out-patient arthroscopy.

WHITWAM, J.G. (ed.) (1994) **Day Case Anaesthesia and Sedation**. Blackwell Scientific Productions, Oxford. Contains a number of scientific chapters which are up to date and readable. Suggests that this is the time for a systematic audit of anaesthesia for day surgery to minimise risk and to promote validated clinical guidelines.

References

BENNER, P. (1984) **From Novice to Expert**. Addison Wesley, Menlo Park.
BUTTERWORTH, T. & FAUGIER, J. (1992) **Clinical Supervision and Mentorship in Nursing**. Chapman and Hall, London.

7

Accountability in Day Surgery Practice

> **THIS CHAPTER:** Discusses the professional role of the nurse and some of the implications and responsibilities associated with nursing accountability. It suggests that professional autonomy, and the greater responsibility which it brings, can reduce risk and maximise effective outcomes in day surgery. It discusses some topical areas of concern to nurses such as skill mix and the scope of professional practice which are important issues in maintaining standards of care. It highlights and gives examples of some common professional dilemmas, which are a consequence of greater autonomy, responsibility and professionalism.

INTRODUCTION

The consequence of educating nurses to a higher level means a greater authority and control of their own area of practice. Another consequence of their 'new' autonomy, though, will be greater accountability for these more knowledgeable practitioners.

This chapter examines some of the responsibilities which are needed for the successful delivery of nursing care in day surgery.

See
Chapter 6 There are some very specific standards of nursing expertise and skill required to care efficiently for day surgery patients, already discussed in the previous chapter. This is because patients spend only short periods of time under direct nursing care, and thus require more support, information and perhaps more confidence than in-patients.

THE CHANGING ROLE OF THE NURSE

There is a fundamental challenge facing nursing today. A number of changes in nursing have come about because of the need to balance the development of scientific and technical skills with the caring or nurturing role traditionally regarded as the primary function of the nurse.

For many years society has placed a high value upon the dedicated, caring and nurturing function which has been traditionally provided by nurses. It has not yet, perhaps, come to terms with the highly skilled, professional and technical contribution which nurses themselves are only beginning to recognise as a large component of their expanding professional responsibility.

Also, in the past, nurses have regarded their main contribution to health care as the 'management of sickness'. Only recently have they been identified as being perfectly placed to take on the preventative, supportive and educative aspects required by a more sophisticated approach to health care (Department of Health 1993). In basic nursing education greater emphasis is now being placed upon the *wellness* of people, on health education and the emerging informational functions of the nurse.

These 'new' functions of nursing are currently emerging as a direct result of changes both from within the NHS, embodied in *The Health of the Nation* (Department of Health 1991), and from society as a whole because of:

■ the changing expectations of patients,

■ greater emphasis upon cost-effectiveness,

■ the need for health education and health promotion within a national health service.

NURSING ACCOUNTABILITY –
or answerability for action taken

Nurses are accountable to a number of different people and organisations during the course of their professional lives. They may, at any one time, be responsible to their medical and nursing colleagues and managers, their professional organisation and, obviously, the organisation which employs them. However, the United Kingdom Central Council (UKCC) Code of Conduct stresses that nurses must be primarily accountable to their patients and this must therefore be their first priority (Box 7.1; UKCC, 1992).

Box 7.1 An extract from UKCC Code of Conduct (1992)

Each registered nurse, midwife and health visitor is accountable for his or her practice and, in the exercise of professional accountability shall:

- Act always in such a way as to promote and safeguard the well-being and interests of patients/clients

- Ensure that no action or omission on his/her part or within his/her sphere of influence is detrimental to the condition, or safety of patients/clients

---

In day surgery, this nursing accountability to patients should ideally extend beyond the boundaries of a hospital visit and the brief episode of care provided within the day surgery system. The important part which each patient plays in their own preparation for surgery and in their post-operative recovery is, arguably, as crucial to a successful outcome as skilled anaesthesia and surgical treatment.

Nurses working in conventional settings have been used to having some control over their patients' progress. They need to feel comfortable about 'letting go' of this control without feeling that they are abandoning their patients 'to their own devices' (MacKenzie Page & Beresford 1988).

Accountability, then, must extend beyond the day surgery experience and a safe and uneventful recovery at home will also frequently require close liaison with community and primary health personnel. If nurses are to extend their responsibility in this direction they will need to provide adequate information for both their patients and their community colleagues.

PROFESSIONAL AUTONOMY: or acting independently, or having the power to do so ('the capacity to think and action one's reasoning – to determine the course of one's own life.' Lee, 1986)

Professionalisation of the nursing workforce lends an exclusiveness to nursing which implies that only registered nurses are entitled to nurse. It can be argued that nursing will never gain true professional autonomy if nursing is carried out by non-nurses. There are, in addition, some important legal implications in using untrained personnel, supervised or unsupervised, to carry out 'nursing' tasks which should also be considered (Harris & Redshaw 1994). These arguments will obviously have implications for all branches of nursing. Therefore, if professional autonomy is to be achieved (as in medicine and law), it should be stated categorically that only qualified personnel will be competent to function as nurses.

It is true that all registered nurses are personally answerable for their practice, and obliged to account for their actions and to justify their professional judgement. However, there should be no problem in employing support staff in day surgery. They can assist with some of the technical skills, within the operating theatre and will take responsibility for 'hotel'-type support such as providing refreshments for patients after surgery and help in preparing them for discharge home. This frees nurses to carry out their primary function as carer and co-ordinator throughout the process.

In the day surgical situation then, although some minor functions within the system may be suitably carried out by support workers and technicians, the unique nature of the educational, informational and supportive role is the responsibility only of qualified nurses whose competence will have been demonstrated through experience and education

See Chapter 6

SKILL MIX: or the numbers *and* skills required for an effective nursing service

It is important for nurses to be aware of the possible consequences of skill mix exercises and cost-efficiency programmes throughout the NHS.

The NHS Management Executive (NHSME) conducted a major review of the out-patient departments in 1990 and recommended a 70% cut in trained nurses. Professor Bevan's report (1989) examined possible redeployment of trained nurses in operating theatres and replacement by operating department personnel.

Day surgery did not escape attention, and skill mix was mentioned (even though it did not form part of their brief), in the Value for Money (VFM) study in 1991. The authors noted the importance of a flexible body of trained nurses capable of working throughout all areas of day surgery, supported by auxiliaries. These support workers could ease the pressure on qualified nurses and would carry out a range of duties appropriate to their grade. It is entirely predictable, however, that administrators will wish to examine cost-cutting in an area where 'minor' treatment is performed. Employing fewer trained nurses and augmenting them with support workers could be a tempting proposition, if prioritisation must be towards the ill in-patient.

However, to refute this, it could be argued that the day surgery nurse is in an ideal position to provide a comprehensive nursing service for large numbers of day patients. Obviously, where professional contact is compressed into a period of a few hours, the importance of skilled support becomes crucial. Although the process of physical care may be only a small component within the day surgical process, each contact between patient and primary (or named) nurse needs to be used for information, education, advice, guidance and support.

SCOPE OF PROFESSIONAL PRACTICE
'General principles or guidelines on which to base changes and developments in the nurse's role, with emphasis upon the benefits to patients coming first' (UKCC 1992)

The report which examined issues surrounding the need to reduce junior doctors' hours has had a considerable impact upon the nursing profession (NHSME 1991). This report not only examined the benefits of other health professionals taking on a number of tasks, previously only carried out by doctors, but also suggested that nurses were in a perfect position to perform some of the mundane tasks which had been the responsibility of junior doctors.

All of the following 'extended roles', they suggested, could be performed by competent and suitably trained nurses:

■ Cannulation,

■ Venepuncture,

■ ECG,

■ X-ray requests,

■ Anaesthetic assistant,

■ Surgeon's assistant,

■ Organising in-patient admissions,

■ Co-ordinating further treatments and follow-up tests.

The nursing profession is having to make some difficult decisions about the appropriateness of taking on these tasks. The pressure will mount, too, as the implementation of the Calman report will have the effect of reducing the service input of junior doctors in training (Calman 1993).

DILEMMAS AND SOLUTIONS

As this pressure increases day surgery nurses will need to determine what criteria they will use in taking on new practices. They will need to weigh up the benefits, in terms of efficiency and enhanced effectiveness for perhaps a few of their patients, against the need for consistent all-round nursing care for all the patients.

The prioritisation and rationing of health care in an increasingly expensive health service is just one of the many issues currently confronting nurses and all health service personnel.

A popular solution to this has been for the government to encourage the expansion of day surgery. Health service organisations are, therefore, being urged to achieve surgical targets in excess of 50% which should be performed as day cases.

This increase in day surgery is obviously of benefit to the health service, in terms of greater numbers of patients being treated. There are, however, some issues (not least that of volume of work and speed of throughput); brought about directly as a consequence of this explosion in day surgery which will concern those nurses who are professionally accountable to their patients.

There are some dilemmas surrounding accountability and adherence to the Code of Professional Conduct (UKCC 1992). These are presented below in a format which highlights some of the problems that day surgery nurses may encounter and with a few possible solutions suggested.

The duty of care – the primacy of patients' interests

The UKCC charges each nurse with ensuring that they *'Act always in such a way as to promote and safeguard the well-being and interests of patients/clients'* (UKCC 1992).

The following dilemmas (which are by no means comprehensive) illustrate some common issues which must be addressed to safeguard the well-being and interests of patients in day surgery.

Common dilemmas

- A patient arrives for pre-assessment who has never undergone a surgical procedure before and does not expect to be discharged before recovery is complete.

- Patients sometimes express concern that their 'minor' treatment entails over-zealous preparation, safety checks and techniques similar to an in-patient treatment.

- A patient may arrive to be assessed for day surgery who displays anxiety about recovery at home, may have severe asthma and/or only their 12-year-old son at home after surgery.

- A patient arrives for day surgery with a history of deep venous thrombosis or other underlying medical problems which they did not consider necessary to mention because of only expecting 'minor' surgery.

Possible solutions

- Ensure, during the pre-assessment interview, that patients understand their treatment, their role in preparing themselves and the necessity for arranging suitable post-operative support and recovery time at home.

- Provide continuing expert nursing care, explanation of the rationale for each procedure, sensory information and constant patient support during all the components of day surgery treatment.

- Inform medical colleagues, after the nursing assessment, of any variations in physical, psychological or social status which may jeopardise safety. Explain the importance of safe selection to patients.

- Select each patient within strict criteria agreed with all day surgery personnel. Formulate these selection criteria specifically to avoid the risk of surgical or anaesthetic complications. Ensure that patients understand these too.

Common dilemmas	Possible solutions
■ Colleagues, agency, bank nurses and managers do not always appreciate the level of skill required to care for patients undergoing general anaesthesia. Staff may be ill equipped to deal with the anaesthetic emergency.	■ Ensure that all staff maintain their competence and skill to provide total patient care and that they are regularly updated in life support technique to cope with the occasional emergency.
■ Some staff expect to transfer responsibility for their patients' support in the community to others both before and after surgery.	■ Ensure that there is a contact point and a day surgery community liaison nurse assigned specifically to provide advice and support both pre- and post-operatively.
■ Priority may not be given to the importance of a multi-disciplinary approach to formulating and agreeing high-quality written information.	■ Consult with the multi-disciplinary team, key personnel and users' groups to provide high quality verbal and written information to patients and their carers before providing a day surgery facility.

Negligence – or a breach in the duty of care

'Ensure that no action or omission ... is detrimental to the condition or safety of patients/clients.' ... 'Take every opportunity to maintain and improve knowledge and competence' and *'acknowledge limitations in competence'* (UKCC 1992).

Nurses are personally responsible for the duties which they have been trained to perform. Since day surgery 'training' is relatively new, it is important to ensure that nurses do not take on any 'extended' roles for which they do not consider themselves competent.

Common dilemmas	Possible solutions
■ Inexperienced staff may fail to inform patients of the implications of their treatment, and particularly their part in ensuring an uneventful recovery	■ Patient information must be consistent, specific and relevant. Nursing staff must have in-depth and up-to-date knowledge about *all* procedures performed in day surgery and the likely effects that patients may experience.
■ Inexperienced nurses may be expected to carry out any of the specific nursing duties which are unique to day surgery without being competent to do so (e.g. being unfamiliar with selection criteria when assessing patient suitability).	■ No new member of staff should perform any task unsupervised or nursing assessment for day surgery until deemed competent . Again, all selection criteria should be made explicit and must be agreed by all the multi-disciplinary team.
■ New staff may be asked to assist with anaesthesia, surgical techniques and recovery without being competent in the specialist skills required.	■ Competence must be acquired in all specialist areas before assisting. It may be useful to enlist support from colleagues in conventional theatres and recovery rooms to help with staff training, because the speed of throughput in day surgery makes time for training difficult.
■ Nurses may be tempted to discharge patients home without being fully satisfied that they will meet the discharge criteria, especially where time is short.	■ Discharge criteria must be made explicit and must be rigorously enforced and agreed among the whole multi-disciplinary team. There must be a guaranteed in-patient bed for any patient who does not meet discharge criteria.

Confidentiality

'Avoid any abuse of the privileged relationship which exists with patients/clients'

'Respect confidential information and refrain from disclosing information without the consent of patient/client' (UKCC 1992)

The dilemma of confidentiality is obviously not unique to day surgery but it is worth considering a few problems which may be encountered by nurses in this setting.

Common dilemmas	Possible solutions
■ A patient asks the nurse not to inform their escort about the nature of the treatment.	■ It is important that *written* information about possible side-effects from treatment is provided to the patient in this case.
■ Nurses may be told confidential information which might affect future treatment.	■ Before confidential information is communicated between relevant health professionals, patients must always be told and should agree to disclosure only to relevant personnel.
■ For a number of valid reasons, some patients may not wish anyone to know about their admission to hospital.	■ These patients must be treated as in-patients since they would have no social support post-operatively.
■ Nurses are not always aware of some of the problems related to access to health records, rights of disclosure and the Data Protection Act (1984).	■ Information technology, computerised records and faxed discharge summaries are subject to the same code of confidentiality as written records.

Informed consent

'the nurse assists in giving patients/clients all the information they want and need to make full and informed choices about their own lives, bodies and health care, ensuring that this information is comprehensible as well as accessible' (Salvage 1987)

Common dilemmas

■ A patient may attend an outreach clinic and therefore does not present for pre-assessment. The nurse does not know if the patient has received all the information needed to undergo the proposed operation and time is short on the day of surgery.

Possible solutions

■ Before the patient receives any treatment or pre-medication they must have the opportunity to discuss the implications with their anaesthetist and surgeon. The nurse must take time to interpret the treatment. An operation may need to be rescheduled to allow a patient to comply with preparation and recovery arrangements.

Documentation and nursing records

'the record is directed primarily to serving the interests and care of the patient or client to whom the record relates ...'.

'the record will demonstrate the chronology of events and all significant consultations, assessments, observation, decisions, interventions and outcomes' (*Standards for Records and Record Keeping, UKCC 1993*)

It cannot be reiterated too often that written records are the only method whereby it is possible to determine retrospectively the relevance, suitability and outcome of day surgical intervention. If nursing documentation is to be effective it will reflect a true summary of all the nursing care provided to the patient.

Common dilemmas	Possible solutions
■ The speed of day surgery treatment makes it difficult to adhere to the standards required for record keeping.	■ All documentation can be prepared in advance with some core care maps to cover those issues which are common to all patients. *See Chapter 4*
	■ Documents can consist of checklists and questionnaires completed by patients. *See Chapter 3*
■ There is a danger that standard care plans are not versatile enough to meet the unique needs of each patient.	■ All plans must be flexible enough to individualise to the special needs and wishes of each patient. Consideration may be given in the future to computerised care planning for day surgery.

CONCLUSION

There will be a number of other dilemmas facing nurses in day surgery which are not mentioned here. However, many of the above will be familiar to most nurses working in day surgery facilities.

It will be apparent from this and from the previous chapters that qualified nurses, experienced in day surgery, can make a considerable contribution to health service efficiency. Their expertise in carrying out patient selection and in providing patient information and education will help to divert suitable patients from in-patient treatment. Without the expertise of nurses, many day patients might be poorly selected, ill-informed and, as a consequence, unhappy with their care.

Therefore, in conclusion, a well-run day surgery facility can minimise the risks of complication and dissatisfaction with the service. Recognising their prime responsibility to patients and exercising accountability, professional autonomy and sensibly increasing their scope of practice into areas where these will be of direct benefit to patients, will all improve standards of care.

ACTION GUIDELINES

- promote the role of the trained nurse in day surgery and understand some of the issues surrounding the changing role of nursing in general

- identify the present level of nursing autonomy and accountability in day surgery and examine the scope for professional expansion in this field

- discuss some common dilemmas in day surgical nursing practice and suggest ways to solve them

Further reading

BALL, J.A., HURST, K., BOOTH, M.R. & FRANKLIN, R. (1989) **But Who will make the Beds?** A Research-based Strategy for Ward Nursing Skills and Resources for the 1990s. Mersey Region Project. A study which assesses nursing staffing and support worker requirements for acute general hospitals.

GREENHALGH & COMPANY Ltd. (1991) **Skill Mix Management, Using Information in Managing the Nursing Resource**. Trent Health. A module of 'the Rainbow Pack' which constitutes a learning programme to manage the nursing resource.

READ. S. (1995) **Catching the Tide: New Voyages in Nursing**? Sheffield Centre for Health and Related Research (SCHARR). Examines the introduction of innovative nursing roles and the issues which have contributed to the pressure for change.

References

BEVAN, P.G. (1989) **The Management and Utilisation of Operating Departments**: A study conducted under the guidance of a Steering Group. NHS Management Executive, VFM Unit.

CALMAN, K. (Chair) (1993) **Hospital Doctors Training for the Future**. The report of the working group on specialist medical training. Department of Health, London.

DEPARTMENT OF HEALTH (1991) **The Health of the Nation**. HMSO, London.

DEPARTMENT OF HEALTH (1993) **A Vision for the Future. The nursing, midwifery and health visiting contribution to health and health care**. Department of Health, London.

HARRIS, A. & REDSHAW, M. (1994) The changing role of the nurse in neonatal care: a study of current practice in England. *Journal of Advanced Nursing* **20** pp. 874-880.

LEE S. (1986) **Law and Morals**. Oxford University Press, Oxford.

MacKENZIE PAGE, S. & BERESFORD L.A. (1988) Planning and documentation - Addressing patient needs in a day surgery setting. *AORN Journal*, **47**, No. 2, pp. 526-537.

NHS MANAGEMENT EXECUTIVE (NHSME) (1990) **The Role of Nurses and Other Non-Medical Staff in Outpatients Departments**. NHSME, London.

NHSME VALUE FOR MONEY UNIT (1991) **Day Surgery, Making it Happen**. HMSO, London.

NHSME (1991) **Junior Doctors, The New Deal**. NHSME, London.

SALVAGE, J. (1987) Whose side are you on? *Senior Nurse*, **6**, No. 2, pp. 20-21.

UNITED KINGDOM CENTRAL COUNCIL (UKCC) FOR NURSING, MIDWIFERY AND HEALTH VISITING (1992) **The Scope of Professional Practice**. UKCC, London.

UNITED KINGDOM CENTRAL COUNCIL FOR NURSING, MIDWIFERY AND HEALTH VISITING (1993) **Standards for Records and Record Keeping**. UKCC, London.

8

A Quality Strategy and the Marketing Of Day Surgery Services

Introduction – The political context – Some definitions – Building a quality strategy – Marketing – Conclusion

THIS CHAPTER: Acknowledges the mounting pressures placed upon health providers to measure the quality and effectiveness of their service. It disentangles some of the jargon associated with some quality initiatives in today's health service to identify them as positive steps in the pursuit of quality of care. It sets quality in the context of day surgery by describing a core set of standards to use as a framework for a quality strategy. Finally, it discusses the concept of marketing with regard to day surgery.

INTRODUCTION

At the risk of oversimplifying what can be very complex issues, this chapter describes some strategies designed to simplify the implementation of a quality programme. It attempts to make the subject more functionally applicable and relevant to the development of high quality day surgery.

The current emphasis on a critical analysis of the health service is designed to encourage the questioning of each component in the delivery of patient care using a variety of audit, research and measurement tools. The ultimate aim is to validate, verify and disseminate 'best practice'. This aim will be achieved by describing those initiatives which are the most cost-effective, responsive and consistently relevant to patient need.

THE POLITICAL CONTEXT

Mounting external pressures and a potentially confusing number of quality initiatives will not have gone unnoticed by those involved in the 'fast lane' of today's NHS. Government policy currently supports and encourages a variety of initiatives, which are intended to encourage and promote efficiency and cost-effectiveness (Lord & Littlejohns 1994). Some of these are listed below.

- Quality measurement through Audit Commission projects

- Central funding for clinical audit

- Research into clinical effectiveness, evidence-based medicine, clinical outcomes and guidelines

- Patient's Charter initiative (1991)

- Financial support for medical research (Culyer 1994)

The consequent challenge to all health professionals in adopting and incorporating any, or all, of these initiatives into everyday practice is a daunting proposition. The situation is probably further complicated by the complexity of the 'internal market' and the formation of new purchasing consortia. These have an impact on every health care organisation within the health service because purchasing organisations are obliged by government to ensure that negotiated performance targets are met by providers.

The methods which purchasers generally use to monitor these targets involves incorporating defined measurable standards and indicators of performance into the quality contracts made with providers. In this way purchasers encourage providers to concentrate on the development of consistent outcomes of care and to demonstrate the effectiveness of their clinical intervention.

SOME DEFINITIONS

Any attempt to disentangle some of the current jargon associated with quality, research methodology and the audit process should start with the translation of these into workable and 'user friendly' definitions (see Box 8.1). Jargon can be counter-productive because it devalues and obscures what should be valuable and valid tools in this pursuit of more effective and consistently higher quality care.

Box 8.1 Some useful definitions

Quality of care: the degree to which effectiveness, efficiency, professional competence, access, availability, satisfaction and acceptability are reached

Clinical audit: applying quality measurement to evaluate clinical issues in order to find out what happens now, which informs what should be happening in the future

Clinical guidelines: research-based methods of clinical treatment

Clinical effectiveness: the extent to which the outcome of clinical care reflects successful treatment in terms of cure, symptom control and quality of life

Clinical outcomes: the measurement and the results of overall clinical performance

Risk management: examination and correction of potential problems within the clinical environment, clinical processes and the competence of personnel to eliminate litigious situations

Internal market: differentiation and formation of purchasing organisations and provider units as separate components within the NHS.

Purchasing consortia: purchasers form large groups to purchase health care by contracting with providers on behalf of the population they serve

---

BUILDING A QUALITY STRATEGY

The following steps are intended as a guide towards developing a quality programme suitable for specific local needs. It is not intended that these should become a substitute for more definitive and detailed examination of quality and the audit process.

The initial approach

There are often difficulties in gaining commitment from the whole multi-disciplinary team. However, this might be solved by introducing the subject into everyday language and avoiding the rhetoric often associated with quality, as suggested in Box 8.1. Defining common goals, agreeing a statement of purpose and discussing the aims of the service will often break down some of the barriers to commitment by drawing the team together. Talking the same language and ensuring a common understanding of what quality really means must be the starting point (Wilson 1992).

Defining the principal functions and objectives of day surgery

The following statements describe some of the principal functions of day surgery. The key words (in bold) are analysed to draw out their meaning.

Statement one

'To provide an **expert, patient-centred** surgical service which is both relevant and accessible to the **specific needs** of day surgery patients'.

'**Expert**' – all staff who work in day surgery are trained in all the relevant and specific components of day surgery. Those in training are always supervised by an expert.

'**Patient-centred**' – the needs
of the patient are paramount.
Staff attend the patient, who
is not expected to fit into
organisational constraints.
Ideally day surgery should be
'a one-stop shop'.

'**Specific needs**' – accurate
selection, pre-assessment,
adequate information for safe
preparation. Process through
day surgery not delayed or
cancelled. Discharge support,
education and carer
information of high standard
and 'user friendly'.

Statement two

'To provide an **efficient** and **effective** service within **finite
resources**'

'**Efficient**' – delays are
eliminated by staggering
appointment times. Staff are
multi-skilled. Lists are
compiled to take account of
recovery times. Start and
finish times are monitored.
All equipment is available
when needed.

'**Effective**' – patients and users
are canvassed for their
opinion about all steps in the
process. Suitable procedures
are selected for day surgery
which guarantee (where
possible) successful outcome
and uneventful, unsupervised
recovery.

'**Finite resources**' –
Unnecessary waste is
minimised or eliminated. All
staff are familiar with the
allocated budget. Accurate
operational costs are
compiled.

Statement three

'To provide a **comprehensive** service which is **responsive** to the wishes of patients and which takes account of the **constraints in the service** and encompasses **research-based practice** and **advances in surgical care**'

'**Comprehensive**' – all
treatment takes place in one
place, where possible. Every
part of treatment is
completed on the day.

'**Responsive**' – flexibility,
ability to adapt to changing
circumstances and the special
needs and wishes of each
patient are catered for, e.g.
family involvement, religious
or culturally specific
requirements.

'**Constraints in the service**' –
limited resources need to be
acknowledged. Staffing,
training and development
limitations, time and
equipment constraints for
more complex procedures.
Delays due to X-ray, laser
availability etc.

'**Research-based practice**' –
the only way to ensure the
efficacy of each day surgery

operation is to measure outcome and keep up to date with new research findings which can improve treatment (e.g. research into new pharmaceutical preparations for anaesthesia tailored to day surgery for quicker recovery; local anaesthetic block for pain control).

'**Advances in surgical care**' – critically examine procedures with debatable benefit to patients (e.g. grommet insertion, D&C), minimally invasive techniques, smaller incisions, image-assisted diagnosis and surgery and laser techniques.

The development of standards

Standard setting is used to assess whether or not a defined level of quality has been achieved. It is the first step in an 'audit cycle' whereby a measurable standard leads to a quality improvement, or a change in practice. The standard will then need to be re-audited to complete the cycle.

Therefore, by formulating a comprehensive set of quality standards against which to measure outcomes of care, measurable improvements can be demonstrated. As shown in Table 8.1, adherence to an agreed level of care can help to minimise some of the risks commonly associated with short-stay surgery.

Obtaining users' views

The term 'user' covers all day surgery 'customers'. The key players who ensure the viability and success of day surgery should all be

Table 8.1 Some standards for day surgery

Standard	Audit
Day surgery waiting lists will be administered and monitored separately from in-patient lists	Waiting times for day surgery Measurement of numbers treated within Patient Charter Standards
All patients will be screened and assessed for physical, social and psychological suitability prior to day surgery admission	Numbers of patients who are found to be unsuitable at pre-assessment: ■ physically ■ socially ■ psychologically ■ inappropriate operation for day surgery ■ patient preference for alternative care
All patients will receive pre-operative instructions and information and will be interviewed to ascertain their understanding, acceptance of and consent to the procedure	Number of patients who: ■ state that they did not receive adequate information and instructions about surgery ■ have not signed consent before day of surgery ■ have not prepared themselves for surgery (e.g. fasted, arranged transport, escort etc.) ■ did not receive information and education from a suitably trained nurse
Patients seen at outreach clinics must receive pre-assessment screening, written postal and verbal information and instructions	Number of patients who: ■ were not screened ■ did not receive postal information and instructions ■ were not given verbal information by clinic staff
Surgery should proceed without undue delay, should not be cancelled or rescheduled	Number of patients whose surgery is delayed due to: ■ poor screening ■ lost documentation ■ inadequate preparation ■ staffing problems ■ poor scheduling, overrunning of lists

Table 8.1 (cont.)

Standard	Audit
Anaesthesia and surgery should be performed by staff who are competent to perform skilled day surgery procedures	Number of patients who: ■ experience anaesthetic complications ■ experience prolonged surgical procedures
The operating theatre should be managed and maintained to provide a safe environment for patients and should be staffed by personnel who are competent in assisting in anaesthesia, and surgical techniques	Incidence where: ■ equipment is substandard or unavailable ■ aseptic technique, theatre safeguards, patient safety and movement is compromised ■ suitably trained staff are unavailable
Recovery from surgery will be managed by suitably trained nurses with all the necessary emergency equipment available	Incidence where: ■ recovery trained nurses are not available ■ equipment is not available or is sub-standard
Pain and other post-operative symptoms must be controlled	Incidence where: ■ pain control is inadequate, inappropriate or not prescribed ■ recovery is delayed due to drowsiness, nausea, hypotension ■ there is unexplained or excessive bleeding or other surgical complication
Post-operative recovery will include adequate supervision and the provision of verbal and written information to both patient and escort prior to discharge to cover as a minimum: ■ details and outcome of operative procedure ■ explanation of normal symptoms and anticipated recovery time	Incidence where: ■ patient and escort express concern about the quality of information provided ■ symptoms and recovery time experienced are not as anticipated ■ pain and symptom control is ineffective ■ follow-up arrangements are not made

Table 8.1   (cont.)

Standard	Audit
■ advice about when to return to normal activity ■ pain and symptom control ■ follow-up arrangements and contact numbers for emergency advice	■ patients and escort are not provided with information in the event of emergencies
Patients will be asked their opinion about their experience and will receive an evaluation phone call to determine progress and outcome	Incidence where: ■ patients describe areas of uncertainty or dissatisfaction with their experience ■ patient is re-admitted ■ process is incomplete because outcome is not noted
Documentation of the day surgery process will cover: ■ pre-assessment screen ■ anaesthetic record ■ surgical procedure performed ■ recovery and discharge criteria met ■ record of information and instructions provided ■ follow-up and further treatment plan ■ outcome and patient satisfaction	Incidence where: ■ documentation does not accurately reflect treatment provided ■ outcome is not noted and satisfaction not ascertained

canvassed for their views and suggestions. Users of the service will include organisations who act on behalf of patients such as:

■ the Community Health Council,

■ purchasers of treatment on behalf of patients,

■ GPs who refer patients to the service,

■ Health care professionals who use the service.

Purchasers of the service, arguably the real 'customers' in today's health service (since they take responsibility for 'buying' health care for their populations), should also be involved at the outset.

They need to be consulted early in the planning process to ensure that their quality standards, targets and views are made explicit and incorporated into the quality programme.

Obtaining the views of patients

The Patient's Charter has had the effect of raising public expectations to such a degree that health professionals are beginning to take more account of the views and wishes of their 'customers'. Throughout this book it has been emphasised that the day patient is expected to take much of the responsibility for their preparation and recovery. This implies the need to formulate a system of consultation with users of the service to ensure 'user' involvement, to determine 'customers' views about the organisation and their perceptions of the quality of the service.

A sample questionnaire to determine patient views is shown in Table 8.2. It can be sent by post to a representative sample of day surgery patients with a request for it to be returned at a suitable time, perhaps 3 to 7 days after recovery is completed at home. Such questionnaires may be of limited use since they reflect the designer's view of what is important. They will also indicate current levels of satisfaction with a variety of issues, but provide little indication of whether or not these issues are important (Morris 1990).

A more extensive questionnaire widely used by the Audit Commission (1991) could also be utilised for a more formal, well-validated method of canvassing patients views.[1]

Complaints

All comments, criticisms and complaints (formal or otherwise) must be taken seriously and investigated thoroughly. Complaints arise as a result of the genuine perceptions and opinions of day surgery treatment seen through the eyes of the patient. They must be regarded as a positive method of improving what patients see as substandard care (Edmondson & Waters 1995).

---

[1] Copies are obtainable from Publication Section, Audit Commission, Nicholson House, Lime Kiln Close, Stoke Gifford, Bristol BS12 6SU.

Table 8.2   **Suggested design for a questionnaire suitable for day surgery**

	YES	NO
Did you receive any written or printed information about your treatment before you went into hospital?	☐	☐
Did you or your escort have problems with car parking at the hospital?	☐	☐
Was your treatment explained to you before you went into hospital?	☐	☐
Did you receive printed information about your operation before coming into hospital?	☐	☐
Did you go home from hospital the same day as your operation?	☐	☐
Were you worried about any of the following? • Injections • Having a general anaesthetic • Your operation • Pain after the operation • Problems managing afterwards • Other (*Please specify*)	☐ ☐ ☐ ☐ ☐ ☐	☐ ☐ ☐ ☐ ☐ ☐
Did you receive enough information about your treatment during your hospital stay?	☐	☐
Did you receive written or printed information about your treatment during your hospital stay?	☐	☐
Did you experience pain during the 24 hours after your operation?	☐	☐
Did you receive any tablets to help with pain control?	☐	☐
Have you experienced any medical complications arising from your treatment in hospital?	☐	☐
Have your symptoms improved since your operation?	☐	☐
Have your symptoms remained the same or got worse since your operation?	☐	☐

Table 8.2 (Continued)

	YES	NO
Since your operation and return home have you been able to:		
• Bathe yourself • Go up and down stairs • Shop • Lift heavy objects • Return to work/normal activity?	☐ ☐ ☐ ☐ ☐	☐ ☐ ☐ ☐ ☐
Have you had to return to hospital for a problem related to your operation?	☐	☐
Have you used any of the following services since leaving hospital?		
• General practitioner • Practice nurse • Hospital out-patients • District nurse • Physiotherapist • Other (*please specify*)	☐ ☐ ☐ ☐ ☐ ☐	☐ ☐ ☐ ☐ ☐ ☐
Would you have liked more help from any of those services since you left hospital?	☐	☐
Have you had to ask for extra help from friends, family or neighbours since you left hospital?	☐	☐
Who was most helpful in explaining your operation?		
• General practitioner • Hospital doctor or surgeon • Hospital nurse • Anaesthetist • Family/friends • Other (*please specify*)	☐ ☐ ☐ ☐ ☐ ☐	☐ ☐ ☐ ☐ ☐ ☐
Would you recommend the same form of treatment to a friend in a similar situation as yourself?	☐	☐

Complaints cannot be dismissed as unimportant on the grounds that patients did not understand the system. Either there has been a breakdown in information supplied to the patient or the staff have failed to ensure that the patient assimilated the information which was provided.

Complaints nearly always possess some element of fact which can be associated with a breakdown in communication and less than adequate information about day surgery procedures and routines. They represent a mismatch between a patient's expectations and what actually did happen.

Every complaint should be analysed to determine:

■ what a patient did expect to experience;

■ why these expectations did not materialise;

■ what actually did occur;

■ what can be done to rectify the mismatch in expectation for the benefit of other patients.

Evaluating quality

The final stage in the implementation of a quality programme is to evaluate whether the objectives and principal functions of the day surgery facility have been realised. This will be achieved through the following:

■ continuous evaluation and research into the outcomes of specific day surgical anaesthesia, surgical techniques and nursing interventions;

■ monitoring and controlling waiting lists and contracts;

■ effective control of allocated resources and by negotiating the re-allocation or redirection of resources to fund developments based on research into the service;

■ monitoring and auditing standards, policies and staff competence through performance reviews, objective setting and reflective practice to safeguard the needs and wishes of patients and their purchasers;

- continuous data collection, research and service improvement, seeking out 'best-practice' and other networking initiatives;

- reviewing and revising policies and standards to reflect more accurately the needs and wishes of the users of the service;

- implementing training/retraining programmes after staff performance review thus guaranteeing appropriate skill levels from all personnel;

- reviewing the usage and continuous programme of maintenance of resources, equipment and supplies.

When evaluating any quality programme it is important to ask whether it is possible to guarantee a certain level of consistency in the quality of the service. This can be evaluated by:

- communication, regular dialogue and feedback between all users and purchasers;

- examining variances, documentation, screening interviews and assessment;

- reporting on incidents and non-compliance in patient selection protocols, assessment, unplanned admissions and re-admissions to hospital;

- the use of relevant research programmes, collection and promulgation of data on all explicit standards and regular reporting of progress in contract performance and service initiatives.

MARKETING

Adopting a quality programme also provides a suitable framework for a marketing strategy. This will be formulated specifically to 'sell' the quality of the service. It can also be used as a basis for negotiation with purchasers and users of the service.

In simple terms marketing involves buying and selling a 'product'. The recent commercial bias in the modern health service has not featured hitherto as a high priority in health care. This has occurred largely because of the advent of the internal market. The aims of any marketing strategy will, therefore, be relatively unfamiliar to most health care personnel. It will, however, become more prominent in all future NHS planning and development, and may be particularly relevant for the continued growth and development of day surgery.

Developing a marketing plan

Costings of day surgery procedures must be made explicit and, while comparisons can be made with similar in-patient procedures, it must not be portrayed as the 'cheaper' option for minor surgery (The Health Business Summary 1993). High quality and extensive communications exercises should be developed to inform and promote the services of the day surgery unit.

Although resources are moving away from the acute care sector, day surgery can be marketed as the preferred option by identifying reductions in the numbers of acute in-patient beds. Thus many future developments can be funded from consequent bed reduction and dis-investment.

A prospectus explaining day surgical services can be formulated to develop dialogues and relationships with:

- patients and the main purchasers of their health care;

- GPs (both fundholders and non-fundholders) as the main referral agencies to day surgery (an increasing number of GPs are forming themselves into powerful purchasing consortia);

- Community Health Councils, Family Health Services and consumer groups.

The important role of individual team members

It is essential that all members of staff work towards making the services of the day surgery unit as attractive as possible to patients, purchasers and their customers. The following points should help to achieve this commitment from staff:

- All staff should be aware of the aims and objectives of the organisation and of their role in publicising these.

- Ambassadors drawn from members of staff can be identified who will promote the benefits and qualities of the unit through road shows, networking and visits. Feedback from these should be systematically collected and analysed.

- All staff can play an important part in identifying issues and concerns. They can suggest improvements to enhance the services of the unit. All collected information will need to be collated, disseminated and appropriate action taken toward the common goal of service improvement.

- Staff must always be aware of the importance of keeping costs competitive and continuous review should be undertaken to eliminate waste and inefficiency.

- Information collected about competitors and their quality of service and initiatives, prices and promotional activity must be obtained, disseminated and analysed to establish if adopting these could be advantageous. Methods of income-generation can be explored and an awareness of new initiatives and achievements in other units should be developed and emulated where desirable.

- Each member of staff must take responsibility for the standard of their verbal and written communication to ensure that this does not conflict with the agreed common goals and corporate style.

- Consideration must be given to all the possible forms of communication with purchasers, patients, visitors, organisations and the public to ensure that timely, accurate and appropriate information is provided.

- Emphasis must be placed on links with the local media in order to raise the profile of day surgery.

CONCLUSION

The day surgery team must be able to identify the changing trends in population needs and purchaser demands, and realise the targets set. By ensuring that there is a quality programme in place and a marketing strategy to sell the service, the image of day surgery will be enhanced.

This will place day surgery in an ideal position to further develop as a versatile and consistently viable, high quality service to an increasing number of patients, which will guarantee the success of day surgery for the future.

ACTION GUIDELINES

- recognise some of the political imperatives associated with providing a quality strategy

- identify the principal functions of a day surgery unit and begin to build a quality strategy based on standard setting and audit of the service

- realise the importance of canvassing the views of all the users of the service

- use complaints as a means of improving the service

- understand the importance of guaranteeing a quality service for effective marketing strategies

Further reading

DONABEDIAN, A. (1966) Evaluating the quality of medical care. *Millbank Memorial Fund Quarterly*, 44, pp. 166–206. An early text which suggested that quality has always been vital to the efficiency and continuation of any process. Organisations must increasingly emphasise quality in their mission statements.

JONES, A. & McDONNELL, U. (1993) **Managing the Clinical Resource**. Baillière Tindall, London. Chapter 8 outlines the role of marketing in health care management and applies some marketing concepts and techniques for clinical practice.

KNUTZEN, B.L. (1989) Ambulatory Surgery, marketing its services. *AORN Journal*, **50**, no. 5. Describes a marketing plan for a Surgi-centre which was designed to improve communication with users of the service.

NHSME (1993) **Day Surgery**. Report by the Day surgery Task Force. Section 3 outlines the criteria for ensuring patient-centred quality assurance for day surgery.

References

AUDIT COMMISSION (1991) **Measuring Quality: The Patient's View of Day Surgery**. HMSO, London.

CULYER, A. (1994) **Supporting Research and Development in the NHS**: A Report to the Minister of Health by a Research and Development Taskforce, HMSO, London.

EDMONDSON, M. & WATERS, G. (1995) Day surgery: handling patient's complaints. *Nursing Standard* Vol. 9 **47**, pp. 25-28.

LORD, J. & LITTLEJOHNS, P. (1994) Secret Garden – clinical audit. *Health Service Journal* 25 Aug., pp. 18-20.

THE HEALTH BUSINESS SUMMARY (1993) **The Economics of Day-case Surgery** (reprint of October 1993 issue).

MORRIS, B. (1990) **Incorporating Customer Requirements in Health Care**, Conference on TQM in Health Care, Birmingham.

WILSON, C.R.M. (1992) **Strategies in Health Care Quality**. W.B. Saunders, Canada.

9

The Future

Introduction – Ambulatory care – The expanding scope of day treatment – Minimal access surgery – Patient hotels – Nursing day patients in the future – An advanced nurse-practitioner in ambulatory care? – Following up care – Liaison between primary and secondary care – Conclusion

THIS CHAPTER: Looks at the future for day surgery and suggests that ambulatory care will begin to embrace more complex treatments within a variety of specialities. It briefly examines the role of an advanced practitioner in the field of ambulatory care and the need to realign boundaries by better communication and liaison between community and hospital. It concludes by urging the nursing profession to be in the vanguard of change in this exciting and dynamic area by pioneering excellent care for an ever-growing number of day patients.

INTRODUCTION

The Royal College of Surgeons (1992) recommended that day surgery should become a legitimate *surgical* speciality in its own right and that it should be performed in a dedicated day surgery unit.

However, as the concept of *ambulatory care* becomes more of a reality, the nursing profession would do well to become more flexible and responsive to the changing face of care in today's society. Nurses must be able to deliver a high level of competent and effective care to all day patients whatever treatment, diagnosis or therapy they may require.

AMBULATORY CARE

Ambulatory care will, in the future embrace a wider variety of specialities and disciplines than is presently the case. The wide variety of treatments carried out as day cases in the future will provide an ideal opportunity to extend and expand nursing's influence into areas previously dominated by the medical profession and the therapies.

Nurses will be needed who can keep up with the changing perspectives surrounding modern ambulatory care. They will need to become rapidly familiar with technological advance and must be confident when working within a number of different disciplines.

The boundaries between what has been regarded as traditional surgical intervention, and the larger numbers of diagnostic, non-invasive and radiologically controlled procedures are becoming increasingly difficult to separate. Day surgery is changing to embrace many 'one day' treatments from a variety of different medical disciplines. This obviously has major implications for nursing since these advances will demand a much more versatile workforce.

Ambulatory nursing care could well become a specialist branch of nursing in its own right with the development of a more extensive portfolio of knowledge, competence and skill to cover many of the areas set out in Box 9.1. In this way, nursing will make a more significant contribution to the future of an expanding system of ambulatory care at the interface between the community services and the acute care sector.

Some definitions

It will be useful here to define some of the new ways in which health care might be delivered in future:

- **Ambulatory care**: Any consultation, procedure, diagnosis or treatment which can be performed within one hospital visit, or a series of visits, and within one day.

Box 9.1   **Expanding areas in day surgery**

■ Extra-capsular extraction of cataract (phaco-emulsification)

■ Pain-control treatments

■ Arthroscopic meniscectomy

■ Radiological drainage of intra-abdominal abscess

■ Radiological diagnostic procedures

■ Laser surgery – prostatic, endometrial ablation

■ Polypectomy, endoscopic biopsy

■ 'Needle' biopsy (breast, lung, liver . . .)

■ Laser angioplasty

■ Retrieval of gallstones

■ Lithotripsy

■ Interventional neurological procedures using spiral CT scanning and MRI

■ **Minimal access surgery**: Surgical intervention usually performed through endoscopic access which reduces the trauma associated with conventional incisional surgery.

■ **Patient hotels**: Facilities provided within easy reach of the place where treatment is provided. These facilities will benefit those low dependency patients who may require further contact with health professionals; who may live considerable distances from the hospital; or who undergo staged treatments.

THE EXPANDING SCOPE OF DAY TREATMENT

It is probably impossible to be truly accurate about the number of day cases presently being treated in Britain today. Some trusts estimated their proportion of day case work for 1993/4 as up to 70% of elective surgery, while the majority estimated their performance at around 40% (NHS Management Executive 1993). There are almost certainly large numbers of day case procedures (not all of which can be identified as legitimate 'day surgery'), which are not accurately recorded as 'day cases'.

Day case patients can be found in nearly every area where health care is provided (see Box 9.2). It will be crucial to collect accurate data on the volume and intensity of day case activity within hospitals, clinics and surgeries if a true picture of the changing trends in health care is to be gained. Accurate data will obviously inform the decision-making process, determine future levels of staffing required and help to analyse the present and future workload of an ambulatory care service.

Box 9.2   Areas where day cases are treated in all the following areas

- In-patient wards as day cases

- Ward attenders for dressings and treatments

- Day wards

- Day surgery units

- Radiology departments

- Endoscopy suites

- Pain clinics

- Out-patient departments

- Programmed investigation units

- GP surgeries

The expanding scope for day surgery treatment

District General Hospitals and Acute Teaching Hospitals are discovering that they will all be expected to achieve higher targets in day case work in the future. Political and financial pressures, rising waiting lists and the current scaling down of acute hospital beds have put the onus on these hospitals to develop innovative approaches to patient care to achieve higher efficiency and reductions in the average length of in-patient stays.

Many surgical procedures which were previously regarded as suitable only for in-patient treatment are now becoming feasible for day surgery. Gradually, too, a majority of diagnostic, laser and radiological treatments are becoming 'in-and-out' day episodes. Although many of these cannot be strictly regarded as *surgical* treatment, they will represent a great deal of the future day case activity in all hospitals.

GP-led minor surgery

There is already considerable debate underway examining the future of minor day surgical treatment in acute hospitals with a view to solving growing waiting lists. It has been suggested that this might be more efficiently performed by suitably qualified GPs in minor-surgery units, 'polyclinics' in the community or in community-style hospitals.

Both day surgery and community nurses should anticipate these future trends and developments. They will need to be 'ahead of the game' as the trend from secondary to primary care becomes a reality.

These trends will change the nature of major acute hospitals and tertiary centres towards performing more of the 'intermediate' surgery. With an emphasis on research, development and training, they will expand and develop their expertise towards minimal access surgery. More of this surgery, with trained, skilled and competent operators, will gradually become appropriate for day case procedures.

There may be a proliferation of GP-run polyclinics taking on a greater proportion of those 'minor' day cases presently referred to hospital consultants. Because of this, practice nurses will need to develop the same specialist skills as hospital day surgery nurses as they begin to provide the same level of care and support for these patients.

MINIMAL ACCESS SURGERY

Patients will in future undergo a number of very complex minimal access therapies and treatments which may not yet be suitably treated as day surgical procedures.

Box 9.3 lists some of the surgical disciplines which are developing their expertise in this area. Boxes 9.4 and 9.5 note some of the advantages and disadvantages of minimal access surgery.

Box 9.3 Surgical specialities employing a minimal access or endoscopic approach

- General surgery

- Gynaecology

- Orthopaedic surgery

- Thoracic surgery

- Urology

- Otorhinolaryngology

- Cardiovascular surgery

- Neurosurgery

A number of 'minimally invasive' treatments have received a bad press in the past because of the poor outcome from a few of the more experimental treatments. Specialist training is offered in a few designated training centres which have been designed to build upon the expertise of surgeons, radiologists and endoscopists (Cuschieri 1993). At present, minimal access surgery is expensive in terms of the specialised nature of some of the equipment and

---

Box 9.4 Some advantages of minimal access surgery

- reduction in post-operative pain
- accelerated recovery
- reduction in post-operative complications
- shorter hospital stays
- earlier return to normal activity
- reduction in wound-related complications

---

disposables required. As expertise increases, however, there are obviously going to be savings in terms of shorter stays, fewer complications and a more rapid recovery.

It is very probable that these patients will require a commensurate level of expertise from nurses specially trained in endosurgical techniques. They will also need guaranteed and consistent continuity of care after their treatment, probably from community nurses who would need to be skilled and knowledgeable about these complex procedures.

Box 9.5 Some disadvantages of minimal access surgery

- high cost of specialist equipment
- more training and expertise required
- few teaching centres available
- poor visualisation of internal structures
- referred pain, absorption of fluid
- longer operation times

PATIENT HOTELS

An overnight facility might be one solution to performing complex procedures which require a certain level of immediate follow-up or monitoring. A patient hotel might also allow day surgery to be performed on patients who may not meet all the strict selection criteria.

The planning and situation of these hotels is crucial to their success. They should represent a 'half-way house' for patients who do not require expert nursing care or observation. They can be situated at some distance from the hospital but should be close enough for ease of access. They should have accommodation for relatives or carers and will ideally be staffed by personnel with some nursing expertise (Value for Money Unit, 1992).

There are a number of patients and their families who would derive some benefit from this facility, but they must be made aware that they *are* hotels or hostels and not hospital wards.

- Those who live a considerable distance from hospital can recover before attempting a long journey home.

- Those who require a post-operative consultation, such as the more elderly patient (particularly relevant to ophthalmology), who can stay overnight for a consultation in the morning.

- Those patients who require staged treatments, such as laser therapy, radiotherapy and more complex radiological treatments but who are not dependent upon skilled nursing care.

NURSING DAY PATIENTS IN THE FUTURE

Because of the more 'major' surgical treatments which ambulatory centres will undoubtedly perform, there is a strong argument for educating nurses to become more familiar and well-versed in every aspect of ambulatory care. Only in this way will the nursing service anticipate and meet the more ambitious targets expected by governments and purchasers in the future.

There must be a consistent and planned approach, by all providers of health care, which is specifically designed to cope with the inevitable shift towards short-stay and day facilities in future. The nursing service needs to keep abreast of new developments, as surgical skill and innovation, anaesthetic and pharmaceutical research gradually transform the patterns of medical treatment. These trends will also increase the demand for more funding to provide adequately resourced integrated day surgery units which can cope with all these new and complex 'high tech' procedures. This may only be achieved, given the finite resources available, by shifting funding from in-patient facilities or from private funding initiatives.

As more patients spend hours rather than days in hospital in the future, it will be important to provide comprehensive, streamlined care plans, shared with and understood by patients, their carers and the primary health team. These care plans must be accurately compiled since they will be used for audit and research purposes to examine critically the way these patients are handled.

AN ADVANCED NURSE-PRACTITIONER IN AMBULATORY CARE?

'The advanced practitioners will provide the continuing advice and support required by the registered practitioners' (Statement from the Working Group comprising UKCC and ENB 1995, cited in Wallace & Gough 1995). The modern trend towards more and more day surgery has already had an impact on nursing practice. There will be a legitimate need, therefore, to extend the scope of nursing's contribution to day case treatments as they inevitably become more complex.

A nurse-practitioner, having undergone higher education and specialised training, will be able to take on clearly identified expert roles and to practise a higher degree of autonomous and advanced nursing care. A possible career path for nurses in ambulatory care could considerably expand the role, widening the scope of practice towards a legitimate 'advanced nurse/practitioner' role.

With a higher level of education and thorough understanding of all the trends in new treatments, the nurse-practitioner might take the main responsibility for:

■ organising and co-ordinating patient care and treatment, providing consistent continuity of care;

■ managing patient assessment, admission and discharge, with the advantage of being personally responsible for keeping patients well informed throughout;

■ providing consistently high standards of nursing expertise throughout all the components of any day procedure;

■ devising and delivering educational programmes and health promotional material, providing support to all categories of day patient and for other nurses working in the field;

■ taking responsibility, and acting as a resource, for follow-up care through liaison and support to patients, community and primary care colleagues.

FOLLOWING UP CARE

In cases where patients and their carers require support and guidance in their own home, day surgery nurses are already beginning to provide advice by means of the mobile phone. After increasingly complex day surgery in the future, patients will probably need more support and information to cope with unexpected symptoms, poorly controlled pain, anaesthetic or surgical complications.

There are a number of ways which will bring community and hospital nursing closer together to guarantee excellent follow-up care. As Fig. 9.1 shows, these strategies can help to break down some of the traditional barriers between hospitals and community services.

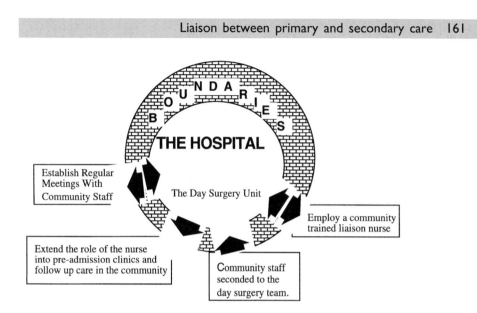

Fig. 9.1   Strategies for breaking down the boundaries between the hospital and the community

LIAISON BETWEEN PRIMARY AND SECONDARY CARE

There are some positive and practical steps which will help to negotiate and realign many of the very tangible boundaries which undoubtedly exist between hospital and community.

Since day surgery nurses cannot realistically be in several places at once, it is crucial that they learn to enlist the support and utilise the skills of the primary health care team to guarantee that there is a continuous process of care. This important contribution from both community nursing and General Practice staff will help patients to feel that there is always someone knowledgeable that they can call upon if necessary.

There is evidence that the impact on GPs following day surgery is minimal where a system of telephone contact from the day surgery nurse is in operation (Jackson *et al.* 1995). Obviously GPs, community nurses and General Practice staff have always been closely involved with the post-operative care of conventional surgical patients. It is important to acknowledge that this involvement is still going to be required regardless of whether patients are day cases or in-patients.

Many community-based staff, however, express a natural anxiety that, as day surgery becomes more complex, they will need to deliver a different level of care to short-stay and day patients which would previously have been carried out during a more lengthy stay in hospital. They report that they find themselves unprepared and inadequately informed when asked to exercise different skills (for example, the removal of drains, pain control, evening visits, regular redressing, support and specific guidance about complex surgical procedures).

Good communication and regular liaison will help to dispel many of these commonly reported anxieties, which can have a detrimental effect on patients if they are communicated between community staff and their patients.

If, however, day surgery is skilfully performed and patients are well-informed and supported, then the increasing numbers of day treatments should not necessarily imply a significant shift from the traditional hospital workload to the primary health team.

The following methods are suggested to ensure good communication and will probably also help to keep the primary health care team fully informed of future trends and changes in day surgery.

Regular meetings with community staff

Probably the best way to allay these very natural anxieties is to develop a mechanism to monitor, support and advise on the problems which community staff do experience. A regular dialogue, combined action plans and policy changes, decided at these meetings, should also help to avoid or solve any problems which are identified.

Meetings or other forms of communication (e.g. newsletters) will keep the primary team informed about new developments, changes in surgical and anaesthetic technique and pain relief strategies which are bound to occur in the fast-moving area of modern day surgery and new day procedures.

Arranging frequent formal meetings is, however, often difficult or impracticable (due to the numbers of different primary health teams in some areas). If they are poorly attended, time-consuming or unproductive, then other strategies may be needed.

Nursing staff secondment

In order to give confidence to community staff who have been out of more acute branches of nursing for some time, it may be beneficial to invite them to spend some time in a day surgery unit. They also bring with them valuable skills for the day surgery nurse to learn, since they help to provide a wider perspective on the holistic nature of a person who is only 'the hospital patient' for a short period of time. Day surgery staff would also benefit from going out into the community to gain insight into the daily lives of their patients and an understanding of the impact which surgery has on their patients.

Employ a community-trained liaison nurse

Employing a community-trained nurse as part of the day surgery establishment might also be a feasible proposition. These nurses would become part of the team and act as liaison nurse for patients, their carers, GPs and practice staff. This may seem to be an unaffordable luxury at present but it should be seen as a natural progression towards the development of a continuous process of care which would enhance the future effectiveness of day surgery nursing.

CONCLUSION

This handbook has described the growth and development of day surgery over recent years. Since the day-to-day management of day surgery unit has generally fallen to the nursing profession to organise, it has stressed the need for meticulous planning and preparation from the whole team. The use of a comprehensive nursing philosophy based on sound theoretical principles should help to ensure a quality service. Accurate selection processes and a multi-faceted nursing assessment, with practical and workable care mapping, will provide a consistent framework around which to deliver excellent care.

Suggestions have been made for preparing protocols and formulating operational policies as an efficient background for managing the day surgery facility. The important part which nurses must play in providing information and patient teaching has been described as have the skills and competence needed for nursing in an integrated day surgery unit, always underpinned by formal education and experienced supervision.

Professional autonomy and the greater responsibility which this brings can reduce the risk of poor outcome. It has also been acknowledged that there are mounting pressures on health providers to measure the quality and effectiveness of their service. To address this, some suggestions have been made for formulating a core set of standards to use as a framework for a quality strategy. Finally, a look into the future emphasises the need to realign boundaries between hospital and community by means of better communication and liaison.

The day surgery nurse is in an ideal position, not merely to believe in a philosophy of 'seamless' care, but to see that vision becoming a reality. A high profile for nursing with achievable standards of nursing competence in all areas of day care is crucially important to the future success of high quality day surgery and ambulatory nursing.

As the future unfolds, nurses should be in the forefront of all these developments. They must retain a firm grasp of their unique contribution in caring for day patients regardless of how or where they are treated. Nursing has a crucial part to play in the future of day surgery, short-stay and ambulatory care and the profession must be prepared to keep pace with the continuous processes of change within this most dynamic area of modern health care.

Further reading

GHOSH, S. & KERSHAW, A.R. (1992) The patient and general practitioners notions of day surgery. *Journal of One Day Surgery* **3** 1, pp. 10-11. A small survey of opinions and perceptions of day surgery from both patient and GP.

VALUE FOR MONEY UNIT (1992) **Patient Hotels: A Quality Alternative to Ward Care**. HMSO, London. Identifies the potential benefits and constraints of accommodating suitable patients in a patient hotel as an alternative to hospital wards.

WALLACE, M. & GOUGH, P. (1995) The UKCC's criteria for specialist and advanced nursing practice. *British Journal of Nursing*, 4, no. 16, pp. 939–952. Examines the development of the UKCC's position on specialist and advanced practice. It considers the evolution of the work within the overall context of post-registration education and practice.

References

CUSCHIERI, A. (1993) **Minimal Access Surgery – Implications for the NHS**. Report from a Working Group, Edinburgh. HMSO, London.

JACKSON, I., DOODSON, M. & HAWKSHAW, D. (1995) A day surgery follow-up. *The Journal of One Day Surgery* 4 no.3. p. 13.

NHS MANAGEMENT EXECUTIVE (1993) **Day Surgery**, Report by the Day Surgery Task Force. NHSME, London.

ROYAL COLLEGE OF SURGEONS OF ENGLAND (1992) **Guidelines for Day Case Surgery**, Royal College of Surgeons, London.

Appendix I:
Current Courses in
Day Surgery Nursing

ENB N33:

Short Programme in Peri-operative and Day Care Nursing Practice for Nurses Experienced in this Field for Nurses, Midwives and Health Visitors on all Parts of the Professional Register working in a perioperative day care setting.

This programme is 10 days in length and leads to an ENB Post-Registration Award. The aims of the programme are to enhance the knowledge and skills of experienced practitioners to provide holistic care in peri-operative and day care nursing, and to facilitate professional development to proficiency level.

Addresses of centres providing N33 courses

Buckinghamshire College, A College of Brunel University, Newland Park, Gorelands Lane, Chalfont St. Giles, Bucks HP8 4AD

Homerton School of Health Studies, Huntingdon Community Unit, Primrose Lane Health Authority, Huntingdon PE18 68E

University of Hertfordshire, School of Health and Human Studies, College Lane, Hatfield, Herts. AL10 9AB.

University of Northumbria at Newcastle, Faculty of Health, Social Work and Education, Teaching Centre, Freeman Hospital, Newcastle upon Tyne NE7 7DN

A21

Perioperative and Day Care Nursing Practice for Nurses on Parts 1 or 12 of the Professional Register

The programme is 24 weeks in length and leads to an ENB Post-registration Award. The aim of the programme is to assist nurses in gaining appropriate knowledge and skills, to provide holistic care to patients/clients in a day care setting.

Addresses of centres providing A21 courses

Coventry and Warwickshire College of Nursing and Midwifery, Administration Block, Walsgrave Hospital, Clifford Bridge Road, Walsgrave, Coventry CV2 2DX.

University of Greenwich, Faculty of Health, Elizabeth Raybould Centre, Bow Arrow Lane, Dartford DA2 6PJ.

De Montfort University, School of Health and Community Studies, Scraptoft Campus, Leicester LE7 9SU.

University of Portsmouth, Department of Health Studies, Queen Alexandra Hospital, Cosham, Portsmouth PO6 3LX.

Kings College, London, Cornwall House Annexe, Waterloo Road, London SE1 8TX.

Kingston University and St. Georges Medical School, Joint Faculty of Healthcare Sciences, 3rd Floor, Millennium House, 21 Eden Street, Kingston upon Thames, Surrey KT1 1BL.

North Yorkshire College of Health, The Innovation Centre, Science Park, University of York, York YO1 5DG.

University of Teesside College of Health, South Cleveland Hospital, Marton Road, Middlesbrough, Cleveland TS3 8BW.

West Yorkshire College of Health Studies, Lea House, Stanley Royd Hospital, Aberford Road, Wakefield, West Yorkshire WF1 4QD.

Specialist organisations

RCN Day Surgery Special Interest Group, c/o Royal College of Nursing, 20 Cavendish Square, London W1M 0AB.

British Association of Day Surgery (BADS), c/o Audit Unit, Royal College of Surgeons, 35-43 Lincoln's Inn Fields, London WC2A 3PN.

Scotland

Professional Studies modules in Same Day Nursing Care

Miss A. Tulloch, Continuing Education Centre, Fife College of Health Studies, Dunnikier Road, KIRKCALDY KY2 5AH.

Mr Matt Winnie, Dept. of Training and Professional Development, Glasgow College of Nursing and Midwifery, 4 Lancaster Crescent, GLASGOW G12 0RR.

Further information can be obtained from:
The National Board for Scotland (NB5), 22 Queen Street, Edinburgh EH2 1NT.

The Welsh National Board: Courses involving Day Surgery

Developments in Surgical Nursing

Department of Nursing, Midwifery and Health Care, University of Wales, Swansea, Parc Beck Campus, Sketty Road, Swansea SA2 9DX.

Advances in Surgical Nursing

School of Nursing and Midwifery Studies, Faculty of Health, University of Wales - Bangor, Fron Heulog, Ffriddoedd Road, Bangor, Gwynedd LL57 2EF.

Mrs J Davies, Assistant Director, South East Wales Institute of Nursing & Midwifery Education, The Grange, Velindre Road, Whitchurch, Cardiff CF4 7XP.

Further information can be obtained from:
Welsh National Board for Nursing, Floor 13, Pearl Assurance
House, Greyfriars Road, Cardiff CF1 3AG.

Northern Ireland

Day Surgery

Southern Area College of Nursing, 68 Lurgan Road, Portadown,
Craigavon, Co. Armagh BT3 5QQ

Surgical Nursing

Western Area College of Nursing, Multidisciplinary Area Hospital,
Londonderry BT27 1SB

Other courses, which have National Board approval, are available
at the Queen's University, Belfast, the University of Ulster, and the
Royal College of Nursing.

For more information contact:
Professor Jean Orr, The Queens University of Belfast.
Tel. 01232 245133

Professor David Sines, The University of Ulster.
Tel. 01265 444141

Mr Michael Bohill, The Royal College of Nursing, Institute of
Advanced Nursing Education.
Tel. 01232 668236

Further information can be obtained from:
The National Board for Nursing, Midwifery and Health Visiting
for Northern Ireland, Centre House, 79 Chichester Street, Belfast
BT1 4JE

Index